DRUGS IN DIABETES

DRUGS IN DIABETES

Editors

Romesh Khardori MD PhD FRCP(C) FACP

Professor of Medicine: Endocrinology and Metabolism
Department of Internal Medicine
Eastern Virginia Medical School
Norfolk, Virginia, United States

Ved V Gossain MD FRCP(C) MACP FACE

Swartz Professor of Medicine
Chief Division of Endocrinology (Emeritus Active)
Michigan State University
Michigan, United States

JAYPEE

JAYPEE BROTHERS MEDICAL PUBLISHERS

The Health Sciences Publisher

New Delhi | London

Jaypee Brothers Medical Publishers (P) Ltd

Headquarters
Jaypee Brothers Medical Publishers (P) Ltd
4838/24, Ansari Road, Daryaganj
New Delhi 110 002, India
Phone: +91-11-43574357
Fax: +91-11-43574314
Email: jaypee@jaypeebrothers.com

Overseas Office
J.P. Medical Ltd
83 Victoria Street, London
SW1H 0HW (UK)
Phone: +44 20 3170 8910
Fax: +44 (0)20 3008 6180
Email: info@jpmedpub.com

Website: www.jaypeebrothers.com
Website: www.jaypeedigital.com

Drugs in Diabetes / *Romesh Khardori, Ved V Gossain*

First Edition: **2021**

ISBN: 978-93-89188-35-6

Printed at

Contributors

Editors

Romesh Khardori MD PhD FRCP(C) FACP
Professor of Medicine: Endocrinology and Metabolism
Department of Internal Medicine
Eastern Virginia Medical School
Norfolk, Virginia, United States

Ved V Gossain MD FRCP(C) MACP FACE
Swartz Professor of Medicine
Chief Division of Endocrinology (Emeritus Active)
Michigan State University
Michigan, United States

Contributing Authors

Aaron B Nelson MD Diplomate, ABIM Internal Medicine, Diplomate, ABIM Endocrinology
Assistant Professor of Medicine
EVMS Center for Endocrine and Metabolic Disorders
Norfolk, Virginia, United States

Ambrish Mithal MD DM
Chairman and Head, Endocrinology and Diabetes Division of Max Healthcare Hospital
Saket, New Delhi, India

Anju Agarwal MD
Fellow in Endocrinology and Metabolism
Michigan State University
East Lansing, Michigan, United States

Arti Bhan MBBS MD
Associate Professor of Medicine
Wayne State University
Division Head
Endocrinology and Metabolism
Henry Ford Health System,
Detroit, Michigan, United States

Andrew Collier MBBS BSc FRCP
Professor
University Hospital of Ayr
Dalmellington Road Ayr
Scotland, United Kingdom

Beatrice Anne M MD (General Medicine) DM (Endocrinology)
Assistant Professor
Department of Endocrinology
Nizam's Institute of Medical Sciences
Hyderabad, Telangana, India

Chaitanya K Mamillapalli
MD MRCP FACE FAPCR
Endocrinologist
Springfield Clinic
Springfield, Illinois, United States

Jacob Moe DO
Consultant Endocrinologist
Associated Endocrinologists
Michigan, United States

Medha Joshi MD
Senior Fellow in Endocrinology
Division of Endocrinology and Metabolism
Eastern Virginia Medical School
Norfolk, Virginia, United States

Parjeet Kaur MD DM
Senior Consultant
Division of Endocrinology and Diabetes
Medanta - The Medicity
Gurugram, Haryana, India

Rajeev Chawla MD FRSSDI F DIAB FACP (USA) FRCP (UK) FACE (USA)
Senior Consultant
Diabetologist and Director
North Delhi Diabetes Centre
Rohini, New Delhi, India

Rana Bhattacharjee
MD (Medicine) MRCP DM (Endocrinology) FICP FACE
Assistant Professor
Department of Endocrinology and Metabolism, IPGME&R and SSKM
Kolkata, West Bengal, India

Rebecca Marie Simon DO
Senior Staff Physician
Henry Ford Health System
Detroit, Michigan, United States

Sailesh Lodha MD (Med) DM Endocrinology (PGI Chandigarh)
Consulting Senior Endocrinologist and Head
Eternal Hospital
Jaipur, Rajasthan, India

Sanjay Kalra MBBS MD DM
Consultant Endocrinologist and Head, Department of Endocrinology, Bharti Hospital
Karnal, Haryana, India

Sarita Bajaj MD (Medicine) DM (Endocrinology, AIIMS) FRCP (London, Glasgow, Edinburgh)
Consultant Endocrinologist
Director-Professor and Head
Department of Medicine
MLN Medical College
Prayagraj, Uttar Pradesh, India

Shalini Jaggi Dip Diab (UK) Dip Endo (UK) F Diab FRSSDI FRCP (London, Glasgow, Edinburgh) FACE
Senior Consultant
Diabetologist and Director
Lifecare Diabetes Centre
Kirti Nagar, New Delhi, India

Sharon Wu Lahiri MD
Clinical Associate Professor
Wayne State University School of Medicine
Director, Endocrinology Fellowship Program
Division of Endocrinology, Diabetes, Bone and Mineral Disorders
Henry Ford Hospital
Detroit, Michigan, United States

Sujoy Ghosh DM FRCP FACE
Associate Professor
Department of Endocrinology
Institute of Post Graduate Medical Education and Research
Kolkata, West Bengal, India

Vishnu Vardhan Garla MD (Endocrinology) MSCI
Assistant Professor
Department of Internal Medicine and Mississippi Center for Clinical and Translational Research, University of Mississippi Medical Center,
Jackson, Mississippi
United States

Preface

With ever-expanding availability of drugs to effectively treat diabetes mellitus, a need was felt to consolidate the armamentarium in a format that would be a readily available resource for medical professionals to choose appropriate drugs. It was felt that a handbook that can be easily carried should serve this purpose. We purposefully stayed away from replicating an abridged pharmacology textbook since that would be unnecessary given the availability of several outstanding textbooks both in print and online. Instead, we chose to offer a catalog that covers the categories of the current available and Food and Drug Administration (FDA) approved medications. We felt that there was no desire to replicate data from any studies since FDA performs a thorough review of studies before a committee votes on approval drugs (majority vote). This was a conscious decision to rely on approval process that is thorough and rigorous.

We believe that we have given our best shot and the product should serve the purpose intended of being a user-friendly reckoner.

This product would not have been possible without the tireless effort of Jaypee Brothers Medical Publishers who kept at it despite many changes of hands at the publishing house. Besides, for almost one year, COVID-19 has created its own difficulties.

While we have tried to observe complete accuracy while writing the book, constructive criticism would be greatly appreciated. We are highly grateful to our contributors for their chapters.

We have taken extreme care to avoid duplication of text. If an inadvertent error or omission has occurred, no responsibility rests with the editors and/or the publishers.

Romesh Khardori MD PhD FRCP(C) FACP
Ved V Gossain MD FRCP(C) MACP FACE

Contents

1

CHAPTER

Management of Type 2 Diabetes Mellitus: A Patient-centered Approach

Sharon Wu Lahiri

INTRODUCTION

Diabetes and its associated health and economic consequences are on the rise with no signs of abatement. The prevalence of diabetes worldwide has nearly doubled from 4.7% in 1980 to 8.5% or 422 million people in 2014.[1] In the United States, 10.5% or 34.2 million people had diabetes in 2018, 21.4% of whom were unaware of their diagnosis.[2] The global direct annual cost of diabetes is estimated to be over 827 billion dollars.[3,4] This costly, growing health problem requires that health professionals become well-versed in treating diabetes and its long-term consequences.

Over the last decade and a half, several new glucose-lowering agents have been developed. Physicians now have a large armamentarium of medications targeting the underlying pathophysiologic abnormalities in type 2 diabetes mellitus (T2DM). The choice of agent(s) to use must be based on patient-specific needs, comorbidities [specifically atherosclerotic cardiovascular disease (ASCVD), heart failure (HF), and chronic kidney disease (CKD)], body mass index and risk of weight gain, risk of adverse effects from treatment including hypoglycemia, ability of the patient to administer and tolerate medications, the efficacy and potency of medications, and cost of treatment.

Excellent comprehensive algorithms on a patient-centered approach to diabetes management have been published by the American Diabetes Association (ADA)/European Association for the Study of Diabetes (EASD) as well as the American Association of Clinical Endocrinologists (AACE)/American College of Endocrinology (ACE) and other groups.[5-13] These algorithms and strategies will be reviewed in this chapter along with a discussion of currently available medications and how to choose among these medications based on patient-specific needs.

PATHOGENESIS OF DIABETES

The "ominous octet" described by Dr Ralph DeFronzo in his 2009 Banting Lecture provides a valuable framework for understanding the underlying pathogenesis of T2DM and the treatment of this chronic disease.[14] "Ominous octet" refers to defects in eight organ systems in T2DM including the liver and muscle (insulin resistance), pancreatic β-cell (insulin deficiency), fat cell (accelerated lipolysis), intestines (incretin deficiency), pancreatic α-cell (excess glucagon production), kidney (increased glucose reabsorption), and brain (impaired appetite regulation and insulin resistance).[14] Therapies targeting the well-known defects of insulin resistance in the muscle and liver [metformin and thiazolidinediones (TZDs)] and β-cell insufficiency (sulfonylureas and insulin) were the primary therapies used until the last decade and a half when newer therapies targeting the other organ system abnormalities became available. These newer agents, glucagon-like peptide-1 (GLP-1) receptor agonists and sodium-glucose cotransporter-2 (SGLT-2) inhibitors, are now considered early in the treatment algorithm in the presence of ASCVD, HF, or CKD due to evidence of their cardiovascular and renal benefits. Furthermore, since these newer medications do not directly stimulate insulin secretion, they do not cause hypoglycemia or weight gain on their own. This is especially important since many glucose-lowering medications are associated with increase in weight, leading to worsening insulin resistance and the need for intensification of treatment, especially with higher doses of insulin, leading to further weight gain. These newer agents can help halt or at least limit the vicious cycle of weight gain from insulin leading to further increase in insulin and weight.

PATIENT-CENTERED CARE

The idea of patient-centered care is not a new concept in primary care. The patient-centered medical home as a model for delivery of primary care was described in 1967 by the American Academy of Pediatrics and developed and endorsed by the major primary care associations in 2007 in the Joint Principles of a patient-centered medical home.[15] Patient-centered care or personalized care in diabetes means taking an individual's unique characteristics, lifestyle, comorbidities, preferences, and abilities into consideration when devising a treatment plan for diabetes and determining how that plan will benefit or adversely affect the individual. An important part of patient-centered care is promoting adherence to the diabetes medication regimen by working to better understand the patient experience with taking the medications, improving the patient–provider relationship to gain patient trust, and obtaining healthcare system support of providers.[16]

Evidence supporting the use of patient-centered care is provided by the DCGP (Diabetes Care in General Practice) study. DCGP looked at the effects of 6 years of intervention with structured personal care versus routine care of T2DM over a 19-year follow-up period.[17] At 19 years, DCGP found that intervention resulted in a lower risk of myocardial infarction and any diabetes-related endpoint.[17] Furthermore, an analysis of a subset of patients with concurrent psychiatric illness from the DCGP study demonstrated that structured personal care resulted in lower risk for all-cause mortality, diabetes-related death, any diabetes-related endpoint, and myocardial infarction.[18]

Several approaches have been published on this topic, all involving the evaluation of the unique characteristics of each patient to determine glycemic goal and careful assessment of the benefits and risks of specific glucose-lowering agents to prescribe a personalized regimen of medications.[5-13]

Glycemic Target

Glycemic targets are determined by weighing the benefits of lower glycated hemoglobin (HbA1c) (reduction in risk of microvascular complications) against the risks of tight control (hypoglycemia, adverse effects from medications, and cost). HbA1c and self-monitored blood glucose levels have been used as parameters of glycemic control, with the former measure being used in most algorithms.

The optimal glycemic target is generally felt to be a HbA1c of 7% or below based on long-term prospective clinical trials demonstrating that tight glycemic control will prevent microvascular complications.[19-22] The UKPDS (United Kingdom Prospective Diabetes Study) evaluated individuals with newly diagnosed T2DM randomized to standard treatment of lifestyle with or without pharmacological therapy to achieve target fasting plasma glucose (FPG) below 15 mmol/L versus intensive treatment with insulin or a sulfonylurea to achieve target FPG below 6 mmol/L over a 10-year period.[19] This landmark study found that the lower HbA1c of 7% achieved in the intensive group (vs. 7.9% in the standard group) was associated with a significant reduction in the risk of microvascular complications.[19] The Kumamoto study also found intensive glycemic control, aiming for a HbA1c below 6.5%, to be beneficial in delaying the onset and progression of microvascular complications in T2DM over a 6-year period.[20]

The impact of intensive glycemic control on macrovascular complications is less certain. A small reduction in risk of myocardial infarction was found with intensive treatment with sulfonylureas and insulin in UKPDS over the 10-year time period, but this was not significant ($p = 0.052$).[19] A significant risk reduction in myocardial infarction, diabetes-related death, and all-cause mortality was found only in a subset of overweight patients in UKPDS randomized to metformin.[21] Interestingly, however, risk reductions for myocardial infarction and death from any cause did become apparent in the intensive group after an additional 10-year follow-up of the UKPDS trial from 1997 to 2007 as more events occurred.[22]

The effects of intensive HbA1c lowering specifically on cardiovascular endpoints were studied in three trials published in 2008: ACCORD (Action to Control Cardiovascular Risk in Diabetes) trial, ADVANCE (Action in Diabetes and Vascular Disease: Preterax and Diamicron Modified Release Controlled Evaluation) trial, and VADT (Veterans Affairs Diabetes Trial).[23-25] The ACCORD trial and VADT targeted a normal HbA1c below 6%, while the ADVANCE trial had a target HbA1c of 6.5% or less.[23-25] The duration of the trials was 5 years for ADVANCE and VADT. ACCORD trial was terminated early at 3.5 years due to increased mortality in the intensive treatment group. The ADVANCE trial and VADT did not find any significant effect of intensive treatment on the rate of major cardiovascular events or death but did find benefit of tight glycemic control on the development and progression of nephropathy.[24,25] The ACCORD trial also did not find a significant reduction in major cardiovascular events, but had an unexpected finding of a 22% relative increase in total mortality, mainly due to increase in death from cardiovascular causes, in the intensive group emerging 1–2 years after randomization.[23] Based on the results of these trials, the general consensus from guidelines and expert opinion is to continue to recommend a HbA1c target of 7% for most patients, although a lower or higher target may be appropriate depending on patient characteristics and comorbidities.[8,9,26,27]

ALGORITHMS AND GUIDELINES

Personalizing diabetes care based on patient characteristics has been recommended by many major organizations. The most comprehensive and widely used algorithms are the position statements by the ADA/EASD, the ADA Standards of Medical Care in Diabetes, and the consensus statement by the AACE/ACE.[7-9]

The ADA Standards of Medical Care recommend determining stringency of glycemic control based on patient preference, risks from hypoglycemia, disease duration, life expectancy, comorbidities and vascular complications, and resources.[9,27] HbA1c goal of <7% is recommended for most nonpregnant adult patients.[27] A more stringent target below 6.5% is felt to be reasonable in healthy patients without cardiovascular disease (CVD) if it can be achieved without significant hypoglycemia or adverse effects of treatment.[27] A less stringent target of

8% should be used in patients with increased risk for severe hypoglycemia, extensive complications and comorbidities, and limited life expectancy.[27]

The ADA/EASD are less specific about HbA1c goals with the algorithm recommending dual therapy be considered when HbA1c is ≥1.5% above the glycemic target based on the aforementioned factors.[7,9,27] Injectable combination therapy with a GLP-1 receptor agonist and/or insulin is recommended by the ADA/EASD when HbA1c is ≥10% or 2% above glycemic target or blood glucose ≥300 mg/dL.[7,9] New in 2019 and 2020 are specific recommendations to use GLP-1 receptor agonists or SGLT-2 inhibitors based on the presence or absence of ASCVD, HF, or CKD.[7,9] In the absence of these three comorbidities, medication choice is based on cost, risk of hypoglycemia, and risk of weight gain.[7,9]

The AACE/ACE algorithm similarly recommends taking patient and medication characteristics into account when determining the glycemic target, but has more stringent goals and is more aggressive with starting and adding glucose-lowering agents. This organization supports a generally lower HbA1c goal of ≤6.5% for most patients to reduce the lifetime risk of microvascular and macrovascular complications, if it can be achieved without hypoglycemia or other adverse effects.[8] Similar to the ADA/EASD algorithm, less stringent control with a HbA1c above 6.5% is recommended if hypoglycemia, comorbidities, macrovascular disease, advanced renal disease, or limited life expectancy are present.[8] Their glycemic control algorithm is stratified based on the initial specific HbA1c level. Pharmacologic therapy with one agent is recommended if the patient presents with HbA1c below 7.5%, while two or three agents are advised if entry HbA1c is above 7.5%; insulin is recommended if HbA1c is above 9% with symptoms of hyperglycemia.[8] This algorithm similarly recommends metformin as first-line therapy and ranks the second- and third-line agents based on the strength of the expert consensus recommendation; those with fewer adverse events, especially weight gain and hypoglycemia, and greater possible benefits, especially cardiovascular or renal, are listed higher, resulting in GLP-1 receptor agonists and SGLT-2 inhibitors having the strongest recommendations.[8]

Other patient-centered algorithms have focused on similar factors for determining treatment. A simple algorithm published in 2010 proposed using four variables (age, body weight, complications, and duration of disease) known as "ABCD" to determine glycemic target and choice of pharmacologic therapy.[10] The Global Partnership for Effective Diabetes Management proposed recommendations in 2010 and 2013 based on similar variables including duration of diabetes, presence of complications, and body weight plus additional factors such as glycemic control over time, history of CVD, and risk of hypoglycemia.[11,12] These algorithms generally recommended targeting a HbA1c close to normal (6.5–7%), if individuals had newly diagnosed diabetes, were of younger age, and had no complications while less stringent targets, closer to 7.5–8%, were recommended for those with complications, CVD, and at risk of hypoglycemia.[10-12] Similarly, Subramanian and Hirsch devised a scale called "Elements of Diabetes Care Scoring Scale" to calculate a score to ascertain the intensity of glycemic control with the goal HbA1c ranging between ≤6.5 and 8.5%.[13] Factors used in this scale include life expectancy based on age, duration of diabetes, glycemic control history, comorbidities, vascular complications, hypoglycemia risk, attitude and diabetes knowledge, and psychosocioeconomic issues.[13]

From these publications and consensus statements, healthcare providers can conclude that stringency of glycemic control and choice of pharmacologic medications should be based on the predicted efficacy, patient ability to tolerate and adhere to a regimen, impact on comorbidities, side effects, and cost.

LIFESTYLE INTERVENTION

Lifestyle therapy is an integral part of diabetes management. If a patient is overweight or obese, weight reduction through dietary means and physical activity is recommended, with consideration of medical or surgical intervention, if indicated. The Diabetes Prevention Program (DPP) and Look Ahead studies have shown that a 7% weight loss is effective in reducing incidence (DPP)[28] or achieving a partial remission of T2DM (Look AHEAD).[29,30] Guidelines recommend weight loss for those with a body mass index of ≥25–30 kg/m^2 through in-person, high-intensity sessions focusing on moderate reduction in caloric intake, increase in physical activity, and use of behavioral strategies to improve adherence to lifestyle changes.[31-33]

GLUCOSE-LOWERING AGENTS

Despite the importance of lifestyle measures, diet and physical activity are often insufficient to reverse or stop the progression of T2DM and the addition of pharmacological therapy is usually necessary. The choice of glucose-lowering agents is based on a patient-centered approach, taking into account: (1) Comorbidities of ASCVD, HF, or CKD, (2) Risk of hypoglycemia, (3) Effect on body weight, (4) Side effects, (5) Cost, and (6) Patient preference.[7,9] Prior to the 2019 guidelines, the decision to start pharmacologic therapy was based on factors such as patient motivation and ability to change lifestyle, predicted efficacy of diet and exercise, and severity of hyperglycemia; Lifestyle intervention could be tried for 3–6 months if HbA1c was near target (7.5% or below).[5,6] New in the 2019 and 2020 guidelines are general recommendations to avoid treatment inertia and aim for more aggressive and rapid titration of treatment to bring HbA1c to goal. A new change in these guidelines is the recommendation to start metformin at diagnosis of diabetes unless contraindications are present, along with lifestyle intervention.[7,9] Evaluation of glycemic status should occur every 3 months with intensification of treatment until HbA1c goal is reached, with choice of treatment being based on the above patient-centered approach.[7,27] The available treatment options, both oral and injectable, target insulin resistance, insulin deficiency, accelerated lipolysis, incretin deficiency, excess glucagon production, increased glucose reabsorption in the kidneys, and increased appetite. This section will provide an overview of the available noninsulin agents for treatment of T2DM and their individual benefits and drawbacks.

Metformin is recommended as initial pharmacologic treatment in T2DM unless contraindications exist. In addition to its ability to lower HbA1c by 1–2% and FPG by 60–70 mg/dL, metformin has the advantages of no hypoglycemia when used as monotherapy, no weight gain and possible modest weight loss, and availability as a generic agent, providing a cost advantage. Metformin reduces the risk of diabetes-related endpoints in overweight patients with T2DM and should always be considered for use in these patients if not contraindicated.[21] The main adverse effect is dose-related gastrointestinal symptoms leading to discontinuation of the medication in 5–10% of patients.[34] Contraindications to its use include conditions that predispose to hypoxemia and lactic acidosis.[34] Renal impairment is also a contraindication, although the Food and Drug Administration (FDA) recently revised warnings to allow continued use of metformin in mild-to-moderate renal impairment estimated glomerular filtration rate (eGFR) 30–45 mL/min/1.73 m^2 if the benefits outweigh the risks.[35]

The insulin secretagogues include sulfonylureas and meglitinides. Sulfonylureas, the oldest class of oral agents, were considered second-line after metformin until the introduction of new agents with alternate mechanisms of action. Their advantages include affordability as generics, efficacy (HbA1c lowering of 1–2%), and proven ability to reduce microvascular complications in T2DM.[19] The cardiovascular effects of the sulfonylurea agents are uncertain. The follow-up study of UKPDS provided evidence of cardiovascular risk reduction,[22] but increased cardiovascular mortality was found to be associated with tolbutamide in the University Group Diabetes Program study.[36] The major disadvantages of the sulfonylureas are the well-known side effects of hypoglycemia and weight gain. Meglitinides are shorter-acting insulin secretagogues administered three times daily before meals. Risk of hypoglycemia is lower due to their short half-life and HbA1c lowering varies from 0.1 to 2%.[37] Due to weight gain and hypoglycemia, the insulin secretagogues are generally not recommended as a second-line or third-line agent unless cost is an issue.[9]

Thiazolidinediones are insulin sensitizers that act as selective agonists for peroxisome proliferator-activated receptor-γ, a superfamily of nuclear receptors that function as ligand-activated transcription factors.[38] Rosiglitazone and pioglitazone are the two TZDs currently approved for use. Benefits include lowering of HbA1c by 1–1.5% and no hypoglycemia as monotherapy. Pioglitazone has been associated with reduction in cardiovascular events, beneficial effects on lipid parameters, and improvements in metabolic and histologic parameters in nonalcoholic steatohepatitis.[39,40] Despite these benefits, TZDs have fallen out of favor for multiple reasons: (1) Side effects of weight gain, (2) Edema, (3) Concerns about HF,[41] (4) Association of rosiglitazone with cardiac events[42] leading to a temporary restriction on its use, (5) Association with bone fractures,[43,44] and (6) Concerns about increased bladder cancer risk with pioglitazone[45-48] leading to an FDA drug safety communication.[49] TZDs can be a second- or third-line agent if cost or minimizing hypoglycemia is an issue.[9]

Incretin-based agents are an important part of our current armamentarium for the management of T2DM. GLP-1 is a gut-derived hormone released from the L cells of the ileum and colon when nutrients, namely carbohydrates, enter the gut. GLP-1 stimulates glucose-dependent pancreatic insulin secretion, suppresses postprandial glucagon secretion, slows gastric emptying, increases satiety, and potentially stimulates insulin gene transcription and β cell growth.[50] In T2DM or impaired glucose tolerance, levels of meal-stimulated GLP-1 are significantly reduced[51] with the extent of change in GLP-1 secretion being inversely correlated with the degree of insulin resistance.[52] Most are given as injections and include exenatide twice daily, two drugs that are given once daily (liraglutide and lixisenatide), and several once weekly formulations (long-acting exenatide, dulaglutide, and semaglutide). An oral version of semaglutide taken once daily was just approved in 2019. Benefits include HbA1c lowering of 1–2% without significant hypoglycemia and weight loss of 1.5–4 kg over 24–52 weeks.[53] The most important and exciting news regarding this group of medications are the recent trial data demonstrating reduction in cardiovascular risk and nephropathy with liraglutide,[54,55] injectable semaglutide,[56] and dulaglutide.[57,58] Albiglutide was also shown to decrease major adverse cardiovascular events but has been off the market since 2017.[59] Due to the impressive and significant findings of 13% decrease in major adverse cardiovascular events (MACE), 22% decrease in death from cardiovascular causes, 12% decrease in nonfatal myocardial infarction, and 15% decrease in death from any cause in the LEADER (Liraglutide Effect and Action in Diabetes: Evaluation of Cardiovascular Outcome Results) trial, liraglutide was FDA approved in 2017 for use to reduce risk of MACE in adults with T2DM and established CVD.[54] Injectable semaglutide and dulaglutide were approved by the FDA in 2020 for reduction in the risk of MACE in adults with T2DM and established CVD based on the SUSTAIN (Semaglutide Unabated Sustainability in Treatment of Type 2 Diabetes) and REWIND (Researching Cardiovascular Events With a Weekly Incretin in Diabetes) trials, respectively.[56,57] The main drawbacks are the concerns about potential risk of pancreatitis and pancreatic cancer,[60,61] C cell hyperplasia and tumors,[62] and gastrointestinal side effects of nausea and vomiting. Semaglutide was also found to be associated with a higher rate of retinopathy complications (HR 1.76), but this does not seem to be a class effect.[56]

An alternate method of increasing GLP-1 is inhibition of dipeptidyl peptidase-4 (DPP-4), the enzyme that breaks GLP-1 down. Four DPP-4 inhibitors are approved for use in the United States: Sitagliptin, saxagliptin, linagliptin, and alogliptin. Compared to GLP-1 receptor agonists, this class of medications has modest glycemic efficacy with ability to lower HbA1c by 0.5–1%, is weight neutral, and does not produce nausea.[63] Pancreatitis has also been reported with use of DPP-4 inhibitors.[64] In 2015, the FDA also issued a warning regarding severe joint pain with this class of drugs.[65] In terms of cardiovascular risk, this class does not have the impressive findings of the GLP-1 receptors agents, but trials showed no increased risk of cardiovascular events or HF with any of these drugs,[66-69] except saxagliptin which was associated with a higher rate of hospitalization for HF compared to placebo.[66]

Sodium-glucose cotransporter type-2 inhibitors, the newest class of glucose-lowering drugs, have a unique mechanism of action that is completely independent of insulin secretion or action. They block renal reabsorption of glucose via SGLT-2 in the proximal convoluted tubule of the kidney.[70] Canagliflozin, dapagliflozin, empagliflozin, and ertugliflozin are the four available drugs in this class. Their benefits include low risk of hypoglycemia, weight loss of 2–3 kg, and blood pressure lowering effects.[71] This class has also been found to have impressive cardiovascular and renal benefits in major trials [EMPA-REG (Empagliflozin Cardiovascular Outcome Event Trial in Type 2 Diabetes Mellitus Patients-Removing Excess Glucose), CANVAS (Canagliflozin Cardiovascular Assessment Study), CREDENCE (Canagliflozin and Renal Events in Diabetes with Established

Nephropathy Clinical Evaluation), and DECLARE-TIMI (Dapagliflozin Effect on Cardiovascular Events–Thrombolysis in Myocardial Infarction)].[72-79] Empagliflozin lowered risk of the primary composite cardiovascular outcome driven by a significant reduction in death from cardiovascular causes, hospitalization for HF, and all-cause mortality leading to a 2016 FDA approval for empagliflozin's use for reduction in risk of cardiovascular death in adults with T2DM with established CVD.[72] Canagliflozin similarly reduced the rate of the primary composite cardiovascular outcome[74] and demonstrated beneficial renal outcomes[75] resulting in a 2018 and 2019 label revision indicating FDA approval for: (1) Reduction in risk of MACE in adults with T2DM and established CVD and (2) Reduction in risk of adverse renal outcomes and hospitalization for HF in adults with T2DM and diabetic nephropathy. Dapagliflozin's beneficial effects on HF led to a label update in 2019 to include use for reduction in the risk of hospitalization from HF in those with T2DM.[76] Based on the results of a new study, DAPA-HF (Dapagliflozin and Prevention of Adverse Outcomes in Heart Failure), in 2020, dapagliflozin became the first diabetes medicine approved as a new treatment for HF in those with reduced ejection fraction (with or without diabetes).[79] The main adverse effect is an increase in genital mycotic infections.[80] Volume depletion and hypotension due to the diuretic effect of the drug can occur but is uncommon, as is acute renal failure.[80] Occurrence of euglycemic diabetic ketoacidosis,[81] an increase in bone fractures[82] and leg/foot amputations with canagliflozin,[74] and Fournier's gangrene[83] have been reported.

Alpha-glucosidase inhibitors are oral agents that slow intestinal carbohydrate absorption through inhibition of intestinal alpha-glucosidase and therefore the conversion into monosaccharides.[84] Available agents in the United States include acarbose and miglitol; voglibose is available in Japan. These agents are especially popular in Asian countries, likely due to consumption of a diet high in carbohydrates, and found to be particularly effective for reducing postprandial glucose levels.[85] A landmark study, STOP-NIDDM, also found that acarbose resulted in a significant reversal of impaired glucose tolerance back to normal glucose tolerance and reduction in cardiovascular events (HR 0.51, $p = 0.03$) compared to placebo.[86] Their lack of popularity in the United States is likely related to the common adverse effects of flatulence and diarrhea.[85]

Two medications used for other conditions, colesevelam and bromocriptine, became approved for use for treatment of T2DM in 2008 and 2009, respectively, but are rarely prescribed for this purpose. Colesevelam, a bile acid sequestrant used for low-density lipoprotein cholesterol (LDL-C) lowering, has a poorly understood mechanism of action with regards to glucose lowering.[87] It is rarely prescribed for diabetes and also infrequently used for cholesterol lowering due to its gastrointestinal side effects and the existence of more efficacious and better tolerated alternative medications. Bromocriptine is a dopamine agonist that is available as a time-release formulation for treatment of T2DM. Its mechanism of action is felt to be reduction in sympathetic nervous system activity, hepatic glucose production, and lipolysis resulting in improved glucose tolerance and insulin sensitivity.[88]

A discussion of the different types of insulin is beyond the scope of this chapter, but differences among insulins with regards to cost, risk of hypoglycemia, and weight gain are discussed below in conjunction with **Table 1.1**.

TABLE 1.1: Recommendations for specific clinical scenarios.

Clinical scenario	Recommendations
Overweight/ obesity	*Preferred noninsulin medications:* • Metformin • GLP-1 receptor agonist • SGLT-2 inhibitor • DPP-4 inhibitor *Avoid:* • Insulin secretagogues • Thiazolidinediones *Insulin*: Detemir has lower weight gain than glargine or NPH[90]
Increased risk of hypoglycemia	*Preferred noninsulin medications:* • Metformin • GLP-1 Receptor Agonist • SGLT-2 inhibitor • DPP-4 inhibitor • Thiazolidinediones *Avoid:* • Insulin secretagogues *Insulin*: Detemir[92] and degludec[93] have lower incidence of hypoglycemia
Renal insufficiency	*Preferred noninsulin medications:* • SGLT-2 inhibitors if eGFR >45 mL/min/1.73 m^2 • GLP-1 receptor agonists if eGFR >30 mL/min/1.73 m^2 • DPP-4 inhibitors: safe at any eGFR; dose adjustment required except for linagliptin *Avoid:* • Insulin secretagogues • Metformin if eGFR <30 mL/min; dose reduction if eGFR <45 mL/min *Insulin*: Careful titration due to slower elimination
Coronary artery disease	*Preferred noninsulin medications:* • GLP-1 receptor agonist • SGLT-2 inhibitor *Avoid:* • Insulin secretagogues *Insulin*: Careful titration to avoid hypoglycemia-HbA1c goal <7%

Continued

Continued

Clinical scenario	Recommendations
Heart failure	*Preferred noninsulin medications:* • SGLT-2 inhibitor • GLP-1 receptor agonist *Avoid:* • Thiazolidinediones • Saxagliptin *Insulin*: Careful titration to avoid hypoglycemia-HbA1c goal <7%
Difficulty complying with injections	*If injections needed:* • Once weekly GLP-1 receptor agonist *If insulin needed:* • Once daily basal insulin with oral agents or GLP-1 receptor agonist or • Twice daily premixed insulin or U500 insulin (if severe insulin resistance)
Lack of insurance or financial limitations	*Preferred noninsulin medications:* • Generic medications: ○ Metformin or sulfonylureas or pioglitazone *Avoid:* • Brand name medications unless copay card available and patient has commercial insurance *If insulin needed:* • Vials less expensive than pens • NPH insulin • Regular insulin

(DPP-4: dipeptidyl peptidase-4; eGFR: estimated glomerular filtration rate; GLP-1: glucagon-like peptide-1; HbA1c: glycated hemoglobin; NPH: neutral protamine Hagedorn; SGLT-2: sodium-glucose cotransporter-2)

INDIVIDUALIZING DRUG CHOICES

A patient-centered approach considers: (1) Patient behavioral and psychological variables, (2) Patient health status and comorbidities, and (3) Characteristics of the pharmacotherapy (see **Box 1.1**).

Specific medications are recommended for certain clinical scenarios as detailed in **Table 1.1**.

The overweight or obese patient with T2DM is commonly encountered in practice. Excess body weight is an established risk factor for T2DM and is often present at diagnosis. Unfortunately, however, these patients are often prescribed glucose-lowering medications associated with weight gain, leading to further increase in weight, worsening insulin resistance, and need for intensification of treatment. Sulfonylureas and TZDs are associated with a 3–5 kg increase in weight. Insulin has an even greater negative effect on weight, causing an average 7 kg gain in weight over 10 years in UKPDS.[19] With regards to type of insulin regimen, a meta-analysis and systematic review showed that increase in body weight was lower with basal insulin than with

BOX 1.1 Patient behavioral/psychological variables, patient health status and comorbidities, and pharmacotherapy characteristics affecting choice of glucose-lowering therapy.

Patient behavioral and psychological variables:

- Motivation
- Level of treatment intensity that is acceptable to the patient
- Acceptance of and ability to use injections
- Treatment history, response, and tolerance to past medications
- Support system
- Food preferences
- Cultural preferences
- Level of physical activity
- Socioeconomic status
- Memory and cognition

Patient health status and comorbidities:

- Age
- Life expectancy
- Disease duration
- Severity of hyperglycemia
- Presence of overweight/obesity
- Tendency toward hypoglycemia/hypoglycemia unawareness
- Macrovascular disease:
    - ASCVD
    - HF
    - Stroke
    - Peripheral vascular disease
- Renal impairment
- Liver dysfunction
- Microvascular complications

Pharmacotherapy characteristics:

- Efficacy
- Risk of hypoglycemia
- Effect on weight
- Side effects/tolerability
- Contraindications
- Effect on cardiac outcomes (ASCVD, HF)
- Effect on renal outcomes
- Drug elimination and clearance
- Cost/insurance coverage
- Oral vs. injectable
- Frequency of dosing

(ASCVD: atherosclerotic cardiovascular disease; HF: heart failure)

a twice-daily insulin regimen or a prandial insulin regimen, although higher insulin doses in the latter two regimens may explain the differences.[89] Weight gain was also found to be lower with use of detemir versus neutral protamine Hagedorn (NPH) or glargine as basal insulin; no difference was found in weight gain with NPH compared to glargine.[89,90] Ultra-long acting basal insulin degludec also does not appear to have any advantage over insulin glargine with regards to limiting weight gain.[91] Choosing medications that are weight neutral or associated with weight loss as initial and subsequent treatment for T2DM in overweight and obese individuals is essential and in accordance with the ADA standards of medical care,[33] the ADA/EASD position statement on hyperglycemia management in T2DM,[7] and the Endocrine Society guidelines on pharmacological management of obesity.[32] The recommended glucose-lowering agents in individuals with T2DM and obesity are metformin,GLP-1 receptor agonists, and SGLT-2 inhibitors for the dual benefit of weight loss and improved glycemic control. Most available evidence points to GLP-1 receptor agonists as being associated with the greatest degree of weight loss.[9]

For patients prone to hypoglycemia, with hypoglycemia unawareness, and at increased risk of adverse outcomes from hypoglycemia, medications with a noninsulin-dependent mechanism of action should be chosen. These medications include SGLT-2 inhibitors, GLP-1 receptor agonists, metformin, or DPP-4 inhibitors.[9] If insulin is needed, insulin detemir and degludec have lower incidence of hypoglycemia compared to glargine or NPH.[92,93]

For patients with CKD or nephropathy, GLP-1 receptor agonists and SGLT-2 inhibitors are recommended and can be used in mild-to-moderate renal impairment. GLP-1 receptor agonists (liraglutide, semaglutide, and dulaglutide) were found to decrease new or worsening diabetic nephropathy.[55,56,58] SGLT-2 inhibitors (empagliflozin, canagliflozin, and dapagliflozin) demonstrated benefit in reducing a renal composite outcome (worsening eGFR, doubling serum creatinine, initiation of renal replacement, and death from renal cause); canagliflozin is approved by the FDA for this indication based on the CREDENCE trial.[73,75,77] Dose adjustment of the GLP-1 receptor agonists, liraglutide, dulaglutide, and semaglutide, is not recommended in renal impairment, but experience of these agents in end-stage renal disease is limited.[94-96] The GLP-1 receptor agonist, liraglutide, has been studied in a small number of patients with severe renal impairment at baseline and not found to have any differences in safety or efficacy compared to patients with normal renal function.[55] Exenatide is not recommended for eGFR below 45 mL/min/1.73 m^2 or end-stage renal disease.[97] No dose adjustment of lixisenatide is required for mild-to-moderate renal impairment, but its use is not recommended with eGFR below 15 mL/min/1.73 m^2.[98] SGLT-2 inhibitors have been found to be effective with eGFR 30–45 mL/min/1.73 m^2,[75] but currently are recommended for use in patients with eGFR >45–60 mL/min/1.73 m^2. Reports of acute kidney injury with SGLT-2 inhibitor use requiring hospitalization or dialysis have also been reported to the FDA, so caution should be exercised and renal function monitored when using in renal insufficiency.[99] The only noninsulin glucose-lowering agents that can be used at any eGFR including end-stage renal disease are the DPP-4 inhibitors. Dose is adjusted based on the eGFR, except for linagliptin which does not require dose adjustment.[63] Metformin can now be used in CKD; It is approved for initiation if eGFR is above 45 mL/min/1.73 m^2, can be continued with assessment of the risks if eGFR falls below 45 mL/min/1.73 m^2, and should be stopped if eGFR falls below 30 mL/min/1.73 m^2.[35]

For patients with CVD, the GLP-1 receptor agonists (liraglutide, semaglutide, and dulaglutide) and SGLT-2 inhibitors (empagliflozin and canagliflozin) decreased risk of MACE and are recommended based on available evidence.[54,56,57,72,74] Empagliflozin and dapagliflozin also significantly reduced risk of hospitalization for HF and should be considered in patients with this condition; dapagliflozin is specifically FDA approved for this indication.[72,79] Sulfonylureas have long been felt to have an uncertain impact and potential negative effect on cardiovascular outcomes based on the UGDP study with tolbutamide and therefore avoided in patients with cardiac disease;[36] however, second- and third-generation sulfonylureas have not been found to be associated with increased risk for death, myocardial infarction, or stroke.[100,101] Thiazolidinediones[41] and the DPP-4 inhibitor saxagliptin[66] should be avoided in HF.

For patients with problems with compliance with multiple daily injections or fear of injections, if injectable agents are indicated, several options with fewer injections are available. Once weekly GLP-1 receptor agonists can be used. If insulin is needed, once daily basal insulin can be combined with a GLP-1 receptor agonist or twice daily insulin regimens can be considered using premixed insulin or U500 insulin for those who are very insulin resistant.

Physicians are often limited in their prescribing by lack of insurance coverage or high copays for brand name medications. In these cases, the oral agents available as generics are metformin, the sulfonylureas, or pioglitazone. The least expensive insulins are NPH insulin and regular insulin.

CONCLUSION

With regards to diabetes management, one size does not fit all. A patient-centered approach is the optimal way to best determine glycemic targets and the appropriate glucose-lowering regimen. The unique characteristics of each patient and each medication need to be taken into consideration when devising the ideal treatment regimen.

REFERENCES

1. World Health Organization. Global report on diabetes. Geneva: World Health Organization; 2016.
2. Centers for Disease Control and Prevention. National Diabetes Statistics Report, 2020, C.f.D.C.a. Prevention, Editor. Atlanta, GA: U.S. Dept of Health and Human Services; 2020.
3. NCD Risk Factor Collaboration (NCD-RisC). Worldwide trends in diabetes since 1980: a pooled analysis of 751 population-based studies with 4.4 million participants. Lancet. 2016;387(10027):1513-30.
4. Seuring T, Archangelidi O, Suhrcke M. The Economic Costs of Type 2 Diabetes: A Global Systematic Review. Pharmacoeconomics. 2015;33(8):811-31.
5. Inzucchi SE, Bergenstal RM, Buse JB, Diamant M, Ferrannini E, Nauck M, et al. Management of hyperglycemia in type 2 diabetes, 2015: a patient-centered approach: update to a position statement of the American Diabetes Association and the European Association for the Study of Diabetes. Diabetes Care. 2015;38(1):140-9.
6. Inzucchi SE, Bergenstal RM, Buse JB, Diamant M, Ferrannini E, Nauck M, et al. Management of hyperglycemia in type 2 diabetes: a patient-centered approach: position statement of the American Diabetes Association (ADA) and the European Association for the Study of Diabetes (EASD). Diabetes Care. 2012;35(6):1364-79.
7. Davies MJ, D'Alessio DA, Fradkin J, Kernan WN, Mathieu C, Mingrone G, et al., Management of Hyperglycemia in Type 2 Diabetes, 2018. A Consensus Report by the American Diabetes Association (ADA) and the European Association for the Study of Diabetes (EASD). Diabetes Care. 2018;41(12):2669-701.
8. Garber AJ, Handelsman Y, Grunberger G, Einhorn D, Abrahamson MJ, Barzilay JI, et al. Consensus Statement by the American Association of Clinical Endocrinologists and American College of Endocrinology on the Comprehensive Type 2 Diabetes Management Algorithm - 2020 Executive Summary. Endocr Pract. 2020;26(1):107-39.
9. American Diabetes Association. 9. Pharmacologic Approaches to Glycemic Treatment: Standards of Medical Care in Diabetes-2020. Diabetes Care. 2020;43:S98-110.
10. Pozzilli P, Leslie RD, Chan J, Fronzo RD, Monnier L, Raz I, et al., The A1C and ABCD of glycaemia management in type 2 diabetes: a physician's personalized approach. Diabetes Metab Res Rev. 2010;26(4):239-44.
11. Del Prato S, LaSalle J, Matthaei S, Bailey CJ, Global Partnership for Effective Diabetes Management. Tailoring treatment to the individual in type 2 diabetes practical guidance from the Global Partnership for Effective Diabetes Management. Int J Clin Pract. 2010;64(3):295-304.
12. Bailey CJ, Aschner P, Del Prato S, LaSalle J, Ji L, Matthaei S, et al., Individualized glycaemic targets and pharmacotherapy in type 2 diabetes. Diab Vasc Dis Res. 2013;10(5):397-409.
13. Subramanian S, Hirsch IB. Personalized diabetes management: Moving from algorithmic to individualized therapy. Diabetes Spectr. 2014;27(2):87-91.
14. Defronzo RA. From the triumvirate to the ominous octet: a new paradigm for the treatment of type 2 diabetes mellitus. Diabetes. 2009;58(4):773-95.
15. American Academy of Family Physicians, American Academy of Pediatrics, American College of Physicians, American Osteopathic Association. Joint principles of a patient-centered medical home. 2007.
16. Schwartz DD, Stewart SD, Aikens JE, Bussell JK, Osborn CY, Safford MM, et al., Seeing the person, not the illness: Promoting diabetes medication adherence through patient-centered collaboration. Clin Diabetes. 2017;35(1):35-42.
17. Hansen LJ, Siersma V, Beck-Nielsen H, de Fine Olivarius N. Structured personal care of type 2 diabetes: a 19 year follow-up of the study Diabetes Care in General Practice (DCGP). Diabetologia. 2013;56(6):1243-53.
18. Larsen JR, Siersma VD, Davidsen AS, Waldorff FB, Reventlow S, de Fine Olivarius N, et al. The excess mortality of patients with diabetes and concurrent

psychiatric illness is markedly reduced by structured personal diabetes care: A 19-year follow up of the randomized controlled study Diabetes Care in General Practice (DCGP). Gen Hosp Psychiatry. 2016;38:42-52.

19. Intensive blood-glucose control with sulphonylureas or insulin compared with conventional treatment and risk of complications in patients with type 2 diabetes (UKPDS 33). UK Prospective Diabetes Study (UKPDS) Group. Lancet. 1998;352(9131):837-53.
20. Ohkubo Y, Kishikawa H, Araki E, Miyata T, Isami S, Motoyoshi S, et al., Intensive insulin therapy prevents the progression of diabetic microvascular complications in Japanese patients with non-insulin-dependent diabetes mellitus: a randomized prospective 6-year study. Diabetes Res Clin Pract. 1995;28(2):103-17.
21. Effect of intensive blood-glucose control with metformin on complications in overweight patients with type 2 diabetes (UKPDS 34). UK Prospective Diabetes Study (UKPDS) Group. Lancet. 1998;352(9131):854-65.
22. Holman RR, Paul SK, Bethel MA, Matthews DR, Neil HA, et al., 10-year follow-up of intensive glucose control in type 2 diabetes. N Engl J Med. 2008;359(15):1577-89.
23. Action to Control Cardiovascular Risk in Diabetes Study Group; Gerstein HC, Miller ME, Byington RP, Goff Jr DC, Bigger JT, et al. Effects of intensive glucose lowering in type 2 diabetes. N Engl J Med. 2008;358(24):2545-59.
24. Patel A, MacMahon S, Chalmers J, Neal B, Billot L, et al., Intensive blood glucose control and vascular outcomes in patients with type 2 diabetes. N Engl J Med. 2008;358(24):2560-72.
25. Duckworth W, Abraira C, Moritz T, Reda D, Emanuele N, Reaven PD, et al., Glucose control and vascular complications in veterans with type 2 diabetes. N Engl J Med. 2009;360(2):129-39.
26. Turnbull FM, Abraira C, Anderson RJ, Byington RP, Chalmers JP, et al. Intensive glucose control and macrovascular outcomes in type 2 diabetes. Diabetologia. 2009;52(11):2288-98.
27. American Diabetes Association. 6. Glycemic Targets: Standards of Medical Care in Diabetes-2020. Diabetes Care. 2020;43:S66-76.
28. Knowler, W.C., Barrett-Connor E, Fowler SE, Hamman RF, Lachin JM, Walker EA, et al. Reduction in the incidence of type 2 diabetes with lifestyle intervention or metformin. N Engl J Med. 2002;346(6):393-403.
29. Gregg EW, Chen H, Wagenknecht LE, Clark JM, Delahanty LM, Bantle J, et al. Association of an intensive lifestyle intervention with remission of type 2 diabetes. JAMA. 2012;308(23):2489-96.
30. Look AHEAD Research Group; Wing RR, Bolin P, Brancati FL, Bray GA, Clark JM, et al. Cardiovascular effects of intensive lifestyle intervention in type 2 diabetes. N Engl J Med. 2013;369(2):145-54.
31. Jensen MD, Ryan DH, Apovian CM, Ard JD, Comuzzie AG, Donato KA, et al., 2013 AHA/ACC/TOS guideline for the management of overweight and obesity in adults: a report of the American College of Cardiology/American Heart Association Task Force on Practice Guidelines and The Obesity Society. Circulation. 2014;129(25):S102-38.
32. Apovian CM, Aronne LJ, Bessesen DH, McDonnell ME, Murad MH, Pagotto U, et al. Pharmacological management of obesity: an endocrine Society clinical practice guideline. J Clin Endocrinol Metab. 2015;100(2):342-62.
33. American Diabetes Association. 8. Obesity management for the treatment of type 2 diabetes: Standards of medical care in diabetes-2020. Diabetes Care. 2020;43:S89-97.
34. Bailey CJ, Turner RC. Metformin. N Engl J Med. 1996;334(9):574-9.
35. Drug Safety Communications (FDA). (2016). FDA Drug Safety Communication: FDA revises warnings regarding use of the diabetes medicine metformin in certain patients with reduced kidney function. [online] Available from: https://www.fda.gov/drugs/drug-safety-and-availability/fda-drug-safety-communication-fda-revises-warnings-regarding-use-diabetes-medicine-metformin-certain#:~:text=The%20current%20drug%20labeling%20

strongly,builds%20up%20in%20the%20blood. [Last accessed September, 2020].

36. Meinert CL, Knatterud GL, Prout TE, Klimt CR. A study of the effects of hypoglycemic agents on vascular complications in patients with adult-onset diabetes. II. Mortality results. Diabetes. 1970;19:789-830.
37. Black C, Donnelly P, McIntyre L, Royle PL, Shepherd JP, Thomas S., Meglitinide analogues for type 2 diabetes mellitus. Cochrane Database Syst Rev. 2007;(2):Cd004654.
38. Yki-Jarvinen H. Thiazolidinediones. N Engl J Med. 2004;351(11):1106-18.
39. Dormandy JA, Charbonnel B, Eckland DJ, Erdmann E, Massi-Benedetti M, Moules IK, et al. Secondary prevention of macrovascular events in patients with type 2 diabetes in the PROactive Study (PROspective pioglitAzone Clinical Trial In macroVascular Events): a randomised controlled trial. Lancet. 2005;366(9493):1279-89.
40. Cusi K, Orsak B, Bril F, Lomonaco R, Hecht J, Ortiz-Lopez C, et al., Long-term pioglitazone treatment for patients with nonalcoholic steatohepatitis and prediabetes or type 2 diabetes mellitus: A randomized trial. Ann Intern Med. 2016;165(5):305-15.
41. Singh S, Loke YK, Furberg CD. Thiazolidinediones and heart failure: a teleo-analysis. Diabetes Care. 2007;30(8):2148-53.
42. Nissen SE, Wolski K. Effect of rosiglitazone on the risk of myocardial infarction and death from cardiovascular causes. N Engl J Med. 2007;356(24):2457-71.
43. Kahn SE, Zinman B, Lachin JM, Haffner SM, Herman WH, Holman RR, et al. Rosiglitazone-associated fractures in type 2 diabetes: an Analysis from A Diabetes Outcome Progression Trial (ADOPT). Diabetes Care. 2008;31(5): 845-51.
44. Viscoli CM, Inzucchi SE, Young LH, Insogna KL, Conwit R, Furie KL, et al. Pioglitazone and risk for bone fracture: Safety data from a randomized clinical trial. J Clin Endocrinol Metab. 2017;102(3):914-922.
45. Ferwana M, Firwana B, Hasan R, Al-Mallah MH, Kim S, Montori VM, et al. Pioglitazone and risk of bladder cancer: a meta-analysis of controlled studies. Diabet Med. 2013;30(9):1026-32.
46. Tuccori M, Filion KB, Yin H, Yu OH, Platt RW, Azoulay L, et al. Pioglitazone use and risk of bladder cancer: population based cohort study. BMJ. 2016;352:i1541.
47. Korhonen P, Heintjes EM, Williams R, Hoti F, Christopher S, Majak M, et al. Pioglitazone use and risk of bladder cancer in patients with type 2 diabetes: retrospective cohort study using datasets from four European countries. BMJ. 2016;354:i3903.
48. Lewis JD, Habel LA, Quesenberry CP, Strom BL, Peng T, Hedderson MM, et al. Pioglitazone use and risk of bladder cancer and other common cancers in persons with diabetes. JAMA. 2015;314(3):265-77.
49. FDA. (2016). FDA Drug Safety Communication: Updated FDA review concludes that use of type 2 diabetes medicine pioglitazone may be linked to an increased risk of bladder cancer. [online] Available from: https://www.fda.gov/drugs/fda-drug-safety-podcasts/fda-drug-safety-podcast-updated-fda-review-concludes-use-pioglitazone-may-be-linked-increased-risk [Last accessed September, 2020].
50. Chia CW, Egan JM. Incretin-based therapies in type 2 diabetes mellitus. J Clin Endocrinol Metab. 2008.;93(10):3703-16.
51. Vilsboll T, Krarup T, Deacon CF, Madsbad S, Holst JJ. Reduced postprandial concentrations of intact biologically active glucagon-like peptide 1 in type 2 diabetic patients. Diabetes. 2001;50(3):609-13.
52. Lugari R, Dei Cas A, Ugolotti D, Finardi L, Barilli AL, Ognibene C, et al., Evidence for early impairment of glucagon-like peptide 1-induced insulin secretion in human type 2 (non insulin-dependent) diabetes. Horm Metab Res. 2002;34(3):150-4.

53. Madsbad S. Review of head-to-head comparisons of glucagon-like peptide-1 receptor agonists. Diabetes Obes Metab. 2016;18(4):317-32.
54. Marso SP, Daniels GH, Brown-Frandsen K, Kristensen P, Mann JF, Nauck MA, et al. Liraglutide and cardiovascular outcomes in type 2 diabetes. N Engl J Med. 2016;375(4):311-22.
55. Mann JFE, Ørsted DD, Brown-Frandsen K, Marso SP, Poulter NR, Rasmussen S, et al. Liraglutide and renal outcomes in type 2 diabetes. N Engl J Med. 2017;377(9):839-48.
56. Marso SP, Bain SC, Consoli A, Eliaschewitz FG, Jódar E, Leiter LA, et al. Semaglutide and cardiovascular outcomes in patients with type 2 diabetes. N Engl J Med. 2016;375(19):1834-44.
57. Gerstein HC, Colhoun HM, Dagenais GR, Diaz R, Lakshmanan M, Pais P, et al. Dulaglutide and cardiovascular outcomes in type 2 diabetes (REWIND): a double-blind, randomised placebo-controlled trial. Lancet. 2019;394(10193):121-30.
58. Gerstein HC, Colhoun HM, Dagenais GR, Diaz R, Lakshmanan M, Pais P, et al. Dulaglutide and renal outcomes in type 2 diabetes: an exploratory analysis of the REWIND randomised, placebo-controlled trial. Lancet. 2019;394(10193):131-8.
59. Hernandez AF, Green JB, Janmohamed S, D'Agostino Sr RB, Granger CB, Jones NP, et al. Albiglutide and cardiovascular outcomes in patients with type 2 diabetes and cardiovascular disease (Harmony Outcomes): a double-blind, randomised placebo-controlled trial. Lancet. 2018;392(10157):1519-29.
60. Butler AE, Campbell-Thompson M, Gurlo T, Dawson DW, Atkinson M, Butler PC. Marked expansion of exocrine and endocrine pancreas with incretin therapy in humans with increased exocrine pancreas dysplasia and the potential for glucagon-producing neuroendocrine tumors. Diabetes. 2013;62(7): 2595-604.
61. European Medicines Agency. (2013). Assessment report for GLP-1 based therapies. [online] Available from: https://www.ema.europa.eu/en/documents/referral/assessment-report-article-53-procedure-glp-1-based-therapies_en.pdf. [Last accessed September, 2020].
62. Bjerre Knudsen L, Madsen LW, Andersen S, Almholt K, de Boer AS, Drucker DJ, et al., Glucagon-like peptide-1 receptor agonists activate rodent thyroid C-cells causing calcitonin release and C-cell proliferation. Endocrinology. 2010;151(4):1473-86.
63. Makrilakis K., The role of DPP-4 inhibitors in the treatment algorithm of type 2 diabetes mellitus: When to select, what to expect. Int J Environ Res Public Health. 2019;16(15):2720.
64. Scheen A. Gliptins (dipeptidyl peptidase-4 inhibitors) and risk of acute pancreatitis. Expert Opin Drug Saf. 2013;12(4):545-57.
65. Men P, He N, Song C, Zhai S. Dipeptidyl peptidase-4 inhibitors and risk of arthralgia: A systematic review and meta-analysis. Diabetes Metab. 2017;43(6):493-500.
66. Scirica BM, Bhatt DL, Braunwald E, Steg PG, Davidson J, Hirshberg B, et al. Saxagliptin and cardiovascular outcomes in patients with type 2 diabetes mellitus. N Engl J Med. 2013;369(14):1317-26.
67. White WB, Cannon CP, Heller SR, Nissen SE, Bergenstal RM, Bakris GL, et al. Alogliptin after acute coronary syndrome in patients with type 2 diabetes. N Engl J Med. 2013;369(14):1327-35.
68. Green JB, Bethel MA, Armstrong PW, Buse JB, Engel SS, Garg J, et al. Effect of sitagliptin on cardiovascular outcomes in type 2 diabetes. N Engl J Med. 2015;373(3):232-42.
69. Rosenstock J, Marx N, Neubacher D, Seck T, Patel S, Woerle HJ, et al. Cardiovascular safety of linagliptin in type 2 diabetes: a comprehensive patient-level pooled analysis of prospectively adjudicated cardiovascular events. Cardiovasc Diabetol. 2015;14:57.

70. Cangoz S, Chang YY, Chempakaseril SJ, Guduru RC, Huynh LM, John JS, et al. The kidney as a new target for antidiabetic drugs: SGLT2 inhibitors. J Clin Pharm Ther. 2013;38(5):350-9.
71. Raskin P. Sodium-glucose cotransporter inhibition: therapeutic potential for the treatment of type 2 diabetes mellitus. Diabetes Metab Res Rev. 2013;29(5):347-56.
72. Zinman B, Wanner S, Lachin JM, Fitchett D, Bluhmki E, Hantel S, et al. Empagliflozin, cardiovascular outcomes, and mortality in type 2 diabetes. N Engl J Med. 2015;373(22):2117-28.
73. Wanner C, Inzucchi SE, Zinman B. Empagliflozin and progression of kidney disease in type 2 diabetes. N Engl J Med. 2016;375(4):323-34.
74. Neal B, Perkovic V, Mahaffey KW, de Zeeuw D, Fulcher G, Erondu N, et al. Canagliflozin and cardiovascular and renal events in type 2 diabetes. N Engl J Med. 2017;377(7):644-57.
75. Perkovic V, Jardine MJ, Neal B, Bompoint S, Heerspink HJ, Charytan DM, et al. Canagliflozin and renal outcomes in type 2 diabetes and nephropathy. N Engl J Med. 2019;380(24):2295-306.
76. Wiviott SD, Raz I, Bonaca MP, Mosenzon O, Kato ET, Cahn A, et al. Dapagliflozin and cardiovascular outcomes in type 2 diabetes. N Engl J Med. 2019;380(4):347-57.
77. Mosenzon O, Wiviott SD, Cahn A, Rozenberg A, Yanuv I, Goodrich EL, et al. Effects of dapagliflozin on development and progression of kidney disease in patients with type 2 diabetes: an analysis from the DECLARE-TIMI 58 randomised trial. Lancet Diabetes Endocrinol. 2019;7(8):606-17.
78. Neuen BL, Young T, Heerspink HJ, Neal B, Perkovic V, Billot L, et al. SGLT2 inhibitors for the prevention of kidney failure in patients with type 2 diabetes: a systematic review and meta-analysis. Lancet Diabetes Endocrinol. 2019;7(11):845-54.
79. McMurray JJV, Solomon SD, Inzucchi SE, Køber L, Kosiborod MN, Martinez FA, et al. Dapagliflozin in patients with heart failure and reduced ejection fraction. N Engl J Med. 2019;381(21):1995-2008.
80. Fitchett D. A safety update on sodium glucose co-transporter 2 inhibitors. Diabetes Obes Metab. 2019;21:34-42.
81. Rosenstock J, Ferrannini E. Euglycemic diabetic ketoacidosis: A predictable, detectable, and preventable safety concern with SGLT2 inhibitors. Diabetes Care. 2015;38(9):1638-42.
82. Watts NB, Bilezikian JP, Usiskin K, Edwards R, Desai M, Law G, et al., Effects of canagliflozin on fracture risk in patients with type 2 diabetes mellitus. J Clin Endocrinol Metab. 2016;101(1):157-66.
83. Bersoff-Matcha SJ, Chamberlain C, Cao C, Kortepeter C, Chong WH. Fournier gangrene associated with sodium-glucose cotransporter-2 inhibitors: A review of spontaneous postmarketing cases. Ann Intern Med. 2019;170(11):764-9.
84. DiNicolantonio JJ, Bhutani J, O'Keefe JH. Acarbose: safe and effective for lowering postprandial hyperglycaemia and improving cardiovascular outcomes. Open Heart. 2015;2(1):e000327.
85. Zhang W, Kim D, Philip E, Miyan Z, Barykina I, Schmidt B, et al. A multinational, observational study to investigate the efficacy, safety and tolerability of acarbose as add-on or monotherapy in a range of patients: the Gluco VIP study. Clin Drug Investig. 2013;33(4):263-74.
86. Chiasson JL, Josse RG, Gomis R, Hanefeld M, Karasik A, Laakso M, et al., Acarbose treatment and the risk of cardiovascular disease and hypertension in patients with impaired glucose tolerance: the STOP-NIDDM trial. JAMA. 2003;290(4):486-94.
87. Fonseca VA, Handelsman Y, Staels B. Colesevelam lowers glucose and lipid levels in type 2 diabetes: the clinical evidence. Diabetes Obes Metab. 2010;12(5):384-92.
88. Defronzo RA. Bromocriptine: a sympatholytic, d2-dopamine agonist for the treatment of type 2 diabetes. Diabetes Care. 2011;34(4):789-94.

89. Pontiroli AE, Miele L, Morabito A. Increase of body weight during the first year of intensive insulin treatment in type 2 diabetes: systematic review and meta-analysis. Diabetes Obes Metab. 2011;13(11):1008-19.
90. Davies MJ, Derezinski T, Pedersen CB, Clauson P. Reduced weight gain with insulin detemir compared to NPH insulin is not explained by a reduction in hypoglycemia. Diabetes Technol Ther. 2008;10(4):273-7.
91. Rodbard HW, Cariou B, Zinman B, Handelsman Y, Philis-Tsimikas A, Skjøth TV, et al. Comparison of insulin degludec with insulin glargine in insulin-naive subjects with type 2 diabetes: A 2-year randomized, treat-to-target trial. Diabet Med. 2013;30(11):1298-304.
92. Strandberg AY, Khanfir H, Mäkimattila S, Saukkonen T, Strandberg TE, Hoti F, et al. Insulins NPH, glargine, and detemir, and risk of severe hypoglycemia among working-age adults. Ann Med. 2017;49(4):357-64.
93. Ratner RE, Gough SCL, Mathieu C, Del Prato S, Bode B, Mersebach H, et al. Hypoglycaemia risk with insulin degludec compared with insulin glargine in type 2 and type 1 diabetes: a pre-planned meta-analysis of phase 3 trials. Diabetes Obes Metab. 2013;15(2):175-84.
94. Novo Nordisk. (2009). Victoza: Prescribing information. Bagsvaerd, Denmark: Novo Nordisk.
95. Novo Nordisk. (2019). Ozempic: Prescribing information. Bagsvaerd, Denmark: Novo Nordisk.
96. Eli Lilly and Company. (2014). Trulicity: Prescribing information. Indianapolis, IN: Eli Lilly and Company.
97. Amylin Ohio LLC. (2019). Bydureon: Prescribing information. Westchester, OH: Amylin Ohio LLC.
98. Sanofi-Aventis U.S., LLC. (2019). Adlyxin: Prescribing information. Bridgewater, NJ: Sanofi-Aventis U.S., LLC.
99. United States Food and Drug Administration. (2016). FDA Drug Safety Communication: FDA strengthens kidney warnings for diabetes medicines canagliflozin (Invokana, Invokamet) and dapagliflozin (Farxiga, Xigduo XR). [online] Available from: https://www.fda.gov/drugs/drug-safety-and-availability/fda-drug-safety-communication-fda-strengthens-kidney-warnings-diabetes-medicines-canagliflozin. [Last accessed September, 2020].
100. Barry HC. Newer sulfonylureas not associated with increased mortality, MIs, or strokes. Am Fam Physician. 2016;94(5):386.
101. Schwartz TB, Meinert CL. The UGDP controversy: thirty-four years of contentious ambiguity laid to rest. Perspect Biol Med. 2004;47(4):564-74.

2

CHAPTER

Second-generation Sulfonylureas

Sarita Bajaj, Sanjay Kalra

INTRODUCTION

The pharmacotherapies available for the treatment of type 2 diabetes mellitus (T2DM) have undergone a dramatic change in the last two decades. Evolution of deeper understanding of the condition at a molecular level and focused research efforts have provided us with newer and more targeted classes of drugs. However, sulfonylureas (SUs) have been used consistently for the past six decades for T2DM treatment, having stood the test of time, considered as contemporary classic in diabetes management. The ancient debate on the safety profile versus the benefits continues to linger on. SUs constitute an important role in the management of diabetes mellitus.

This chapter aims to discuss the historical aspects and the evolution of role of SU as front runners in management of hyperglycemia along with their mechanism of action, safety profile and adverse effects.

HISTORY

It was until 1950s that insulin remained the only pharmacological treatment for type 1 diabetes mellitus (T1DM) and T2DM patients. Then a paradigm shift in the treatment of diabetes was a result of serendipity traced back to 1942 when Marcel Janbon, an infectious disease physician while experimenting with a new sulfonamide for treatment of typhoid fever, shared his findings of post-treatment convulsions, prolonged coma, and significant drop in blood glucose in some of the patients to his physiologist colleague Auguste-Louis Loubatières, who had been conducting diabetes research in dogs during the previous decade. Later Loubatières, after a series of research work, concluded that sulfonamide was an insulin secretagogue acting directly on the pancreas.[1] But it was not until 1956 that the first sulfonylurea, tolbutamide, was introduced commercially in Germany.[2]

TABLE 2.1: **Classification of sulfonylureas.**

First-generation sulfonylureas	• Tolbutamide • Acetohexamide • Tolazamide • Chlorpropamide
Second-generation sulfonylureas • Conventional • Modern	• Glibenclamide • Glipizide • Glimepiride • Gliclazide • Gliclazide MR, XR • Glipizide XL

(MR: modified release; XR/XL: extended release)

FIRST-GENERATION SULFONYLUREAS

Four drugs, namely, tolbutamide, acetohexamide, tolazamide, and chlorpropamide, were commonly being prescribed by mid-1960s (**Table 2.1**). All these had distinct pharmacokinetics and pharmacodynamics. Nevertheless, the University Group Diabetes Program (UGDP)[3] performed a study over an extended period to observe the efficiency of tolbutamide, phenformin, and insulin. The initial results showed inefficiency and high susceptibility of cardiovascular (CV) mortality with of tolbutamide. As a result, the clinical prescription of these drugs came down substantially and diet modification and/or insulin was considered the treatment of choice.

The successive presentation of errors in UGDP observations and the rejection or disapproval of the results by the American Diabetes Association (ADA), apart from contrasting results obtained by various other researches, generated the establishment of these drugs in clinical use globally. However, the US Food and Drug Administration (USFDA) insists on adding warning insert regarding the increased susceptibility to CV comorbidities in the package of these agents.[4]

SECOND-GENERATION SULFONYLUREAS

Subsequently second-generation SUs, i.e., glipizide, glibenclamide, gliclazide, and glimepiride became available (**Table 2.2**). Glyburide and glipizide were first introduced in Europe for several years before becoming available in the United States in 1984.[4] Glimepiride became the latest second-generation SU to be introduced into clinical practice, first in Sweden and then subsequently got USFDA approval in 1995.[5]

All SUs have been shown to trigger insulin production and probably have the potential to regulate blood glucose in the absence of considerably stimulated production of insulin. This led to the hypothesis that SUs acted on two sites: Firstly, in the β-cell membrane and the next in an unspecified extrapancreatic site. Though it was accepted that SUs reduced blood glucose

TABLE 2.2: Characteristics of second-generation sulfonylureas (SU).

SU	Daily dose	Duration of action	Dose in renal failure	Dose in hepatic failure	Ischemic preconditioning
Glibenclamide	1.25–20 mg, single or two divided doses	16–24 h	Not recommended in CrCl <50 mL/min	Avoid in severe cases	Abolished
Glimepiride	1–8 mg, single dose	24 h	Reduce, start at 1 mg	Avoid in severe cases	Preserved
Gliclazide	40–320 mg, single or divided doses	10–24 h	No dose adjustment	Avoid in severe cases	Preserved
Gliclazide MR/XR	30–120 mg, single dose	>24 h	No dose adjustment	Avoid in severe cases	Preserved
Glipizide	2.5–40 mg, single or two divided doses	12–24 h	No dose adjustment	Reduce, start at 2.5 mg	Preserved
Glipizide XL	5–20 mg, single dose	>24 h	No dose adjustment	Reduce, start at 2.5 mg	Preserved

(CrCl: creatinine clearance; MR: modified release; XR/XL: extended release) level, the mechanism by which this action occurred remained to be elucidated. In 1984, ATP sensitive potassium channel (K_{ATP}) was identified in pancreatic islets. Later in 1995, the precise binding area for SU, Subunit sulfonylurea receptor 1 (SUR1), on the ATP sensitive potassium channel was reported.[6]

Evidence from literature suggests that SUs account for up to 20% of newly initiated oral antidiabetic drugs (OADs), either as monotherapy or in combination, for the treatment of T2DM presumably because they are relatively inexpensive, allow for once-daily oral dosing (in some cases), have reliable efficacy in reducing blood-glucose, and rarely cause symptomatic side effects other than hypoglycemia and weight gain. More than 40 years after the UGDP, their risks versus benefits are still debated.[7] Some SUs are believed to accelerate β-cell apoptosis, increase the risk of ischemic complications, and contribute to nonfatal CV outcomes and all-cause mortality.[8]

However, with the availability of modern second-generation SUs with fewer side effects and better efficacy, their popularity has not waned. A patient centered approach which includes careful selection of SU, the appropriate dosage, proper timing of administration, and adequate patient counseling will ensure that deserving patients are not deprived of the advantages of this well-established class of OADs.[8]

PHARMACOLOGY: MECHANISM OF ACTION

Sulfonylureas are classified as insulin secretagogues (**Fig. 2.1**). They trigger endogenous insulin production by limiting the K_{ATPs} located on pancreatic β-cells. They attach to the SUR subunit located on the β-cell plasma membrane and lead to K_{ATP} channel closing and stop efflux of K^+. Further, the membrane is depolarized thereby allowing influx of Ca^{2+} ions. Finally, this causes stimulation of insulin secretion from secretory vesicles. As production of insulin is a glucose-mediated activity, the regular SUs are analogous with an increased susceptibility of hypoglycemia.[8]

ARE ALL SULFONYLUREAS THE SAME?

Sulfonylureas stimulate insulin secretion by blocking K_{ATP} channels in the pancreatic β-cell membrane by binding to the SUR subunit of the channel. K_{ATP} channels are also present at extra pancreatic tissues, but often contain different types of SUR subunit. Recent evidences suggest that there are variations in the effect of SU on these K_{ATP} channels located in different tissues. For example, tolbutamide and gliclazide block SUR1 with higher affinity as compared to SUR2 while glimepiride and glibenclamide block both SUR1 and SUR2 receptors with similar affinity. The reversibility property shows differences

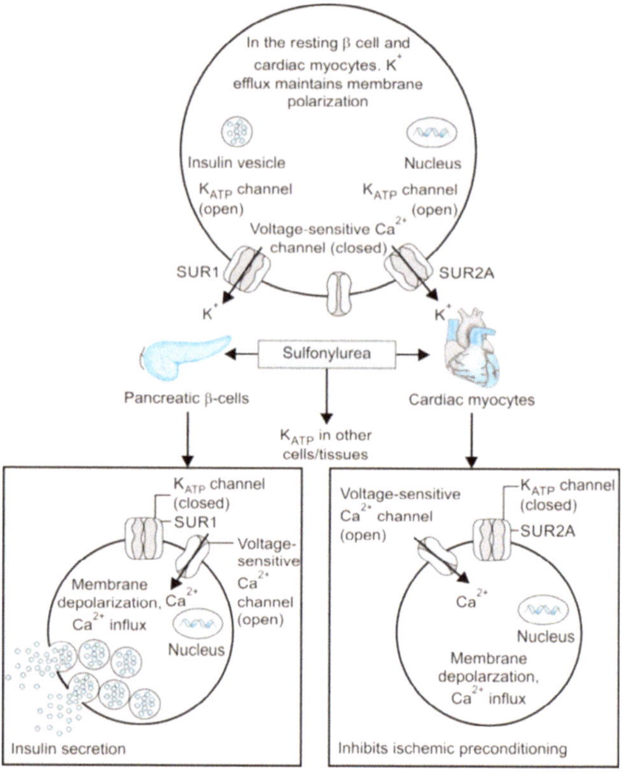

(SUR1: sulfonylurea receptor 1)

FIG. 2.1: Mechanism of action of sulfonylurea.

Source: Adapted from Kalra S, Aamir AH, Raza A, Das AK, Khan AK, Shrestha D, et al. Place of SU in the management of type 2 diabetes mellitus in South Asia: a consensus statement. Indian J Endocr Metab. 2015;19:577-96.

between the agents. On one hand, tolbutamide and gliclazide cause a reversible inhibition of Kir6.2/SUR1 and Kir6.2/SUR2 channels. On the other hand, the cardiac action of glibenclamide is reversible while β-cell, K_{ATP} channels are not reversible. Particularly, SUs that impede SUR1 reversibly (tolbutamide and gliclazide) have lesser number of hydrophobic groups than SUs that are gradually reversible (glibenclamide and glimepiride). The differences can possibly be described by taking into account the hetero-octameric complex of SUR1-K_{ATP} channels that have two high-affinity attachment sites for sulfonyl moiety and benzamido moiety, respectively. The selectivity of SUR1 for the sulfonyl moiety is 100 to 1,000-folds more than that for SUR2. Nearly, all SUs have both sulfonyl and benzamido moieties and interact with SUR1 and SUR2. In contrast, short-chain molecules as in gliclazide attach specifically to sulfonyl site and have no benzamido moiety. This substantiates the selectivity of short-chain SU such as gliclazide by the pancreas partly. Glimepiride triggers insulin production by attaching to precisely 65kD a protein site on the K_{ATP} channel of pancreatic β-cell and applies allosteric inhibition of the SUR complex. When contrasted with glibenclamide, glimepiride shows lesser binding affinity (2 to 3-fold) for SUR and more chances of association (2.5 to 3-fold) and dissociation (8 to 9-fold) from the receptor. The specific binding site and receptor associations of glimepiride are supposed to produce lesser inhibition of K_{ATP} channel and therefore the proneness to hypoglycemia is reduced. In addition, the potential of glimepiride to increase both phases of insulin production in T2DM subjects shows a probable association between optimal glycemic control and drastic improvement of regularity of in vivo insulin secretory function. All second-generation SUs except gliclazide are shown to bind to Epac2, a triggering stimulus for insulin exocytosis. As a result, with gliclazide there is lesser susceptibility of hypoglycemia. The changes in pharmacodynamic/pharmacokinetic (PD/PK) profiles of the specific SUs suggest the distinctions in antidiabetic activity, proneness to hypoglycemia, specificities to multiple tissue specific SURs, influence on myocardial ischemic preconditioning, and insulin secretory factors. Taking these factors into consideration it is better to choose from newer second-generation SUs.[8]

GLYCEMIC EFFICACY

Second-generation SUs have shown a robust evidence for glycemic lowering, both as monotherapy and in combination with other OADs. In a recent systemic review and meta-analysis, SU monotherapy was found to reduce glycated hemoglobin (HbA1c) by 1.51% as compared to placebo. HbA1c reduction and improvement in long-term outcome from intensive glycemic control with SU-based therapies that have been established by numerous significant studies including the UKPDS (United Kingdom Prospective Diabetes Study), the ADVANCE (Action in Diabetes and Vascular Disease: Preterax and Diamicron Modified-release Controlled Evaluation), the ADOPT (A Diabetes Outcome Progression Trial), and the VADTFS (Veterans Affairs Diabetes Trial Follow-up Study).[8]

EFFICACY REGARDING MICROVASCULAR AND MACROVASCULAR COMPLICATIONS

The UKPDS[9] and ADVANCE[10] trials showed an improved long-term outcome with sulfonylurea-based intensive therapy. A 10-year follow-up of UKPDS suggested that intensive control with either insulin or SU was associated with relative risk (RR) reductions of 9% in diabetes-related end point, 24% in microvascular disease, and 15% for myocardial infarction and 13% in death from any cause. In the ADVANCE trial, the strategy of intensive glucose control targeting HbA1c under 6.5% involving gliclazide (modified release) reduced the average HbA1c value to 6.5 % in a wider range of patients with T2DM and had significantly reduced the incidence of the combined primary outcome of major macrovascular or microvascular events (i.e., 18.1% in the intensive control group vs. 20.0% in the standard control group). The main contributor to the 10% relative reduction in the primary outcome found with intensive control as compared with standard control was a 21% relative reduction in the risk of new or worsening nephropathy. Also, there was significant reduction in major microvascular events (9.4% in intensive control group vs. 10.9% in the standard control group) without any unfavorable CV outcomes. However, no evidence of a reduction in macrovascular events was found. Additionally, a 10% reduction in risk of serious diabetes complications and 30% in macroalbuminuria development was observed in patients in intensive control group. Similarly, in the ADVANCE-ON study,[11] which used intensive target driven multifactorial approach with SU therapy, the reduction in the risk of microvascular complications (specifically end stage renal disease) was observed. On similar lines, 10-year results of VADTFS[12] demonstrated that intensive treatment results in a 17% relative reduction in major CV events compared to standard care, with no difference in mortality.[8]

ADVERSE EFFECTS

Adverse effects, other than hypoglycemia and weight gain, with the use of modern second-generation SUs include symptomatic hyponatremia, alcohol induced flushing or disulfiram-like reaction, cholestatic jaundice, macular erythema, rash, and blood dyscrasias. Conventional SU may be associated with dizziness and headache, hyponatremia, anemia, leukopenia, and thrombocytopenia.[8]

EXTRAPANCREATIC EFFECTS

Sulfonylureas have insulin sensitizing action by elevating the release of glucose transporter type 4 (GLUT4) transporters and reducing resistance of insulin in peripheral tissues. SUs have a CV influence regulated by impeding sarcolemmal and mitochondrial K_{ATP} channels located on cardiac myocytes and K_{ATP} channels situated on vascular smooth muscle cell. The consequence of this action is the damage of ischemic preconditioning (IPC), a cardioprotective phenomenon. Still glimepiride did not harm IPC, though it showed anti-inflammatory and angiogenic activity inT2DM subjects. Also, an antioxidative and provascular influence is seen with glimepiride due to its reduced toxic advanced glycation end products (AGEs) and soluble receptor for AGE (sRAGE) and elevated colony stimulating factors.[8]

Gliclazide applies its extrapancreatic actions by strengthening insulin mediated glucose uptake in muscles (+35%) to elevate insulin sensitivity. These influences are in harmony with post-transcriptional function of gliclazide on GLUT4 transporters. It has been observed that gliclazide decreases hepatic glucose secretion and enhances fasting glycemia. The actions of gliclazide include endovascular and antioxidant actions.

- Reducing microthrombosis through partial inhibition of platelet aggregation/adhesion.
- Elevating vascular endothelium fibrinolytic activity.
- Reducing plasma lipid peroxide.
- Increasing erythrocyte superoxide dismutase.[8]

SECOND-GENERATION SULFONYLUREAS: APPLIED ASPECTS

Beta-cell Apoptosis

Concerns are raised by investigators regarding SU-induced β-cell exhaustion, although the data remains largely inconsistent.[13] Exposure of glibenclamide in cultured human islet cell was found to induce apoptosis.[14] The UKPDS and ADOPT trials also implicated glibenclamide for secondary failure in majority of patients after an effective initial response.[8] However, the data from a systemic review of three RCTs presented a contrasting picture with gliclazide showing lower rates of secondary failure of 7.0% as compared to glibenclamide 17.9% ($p < 0.1$) and glipizide 25.6% ($p < 0.005$), respectively. Potential mechanisms suggested for β-cell apoptosis are sustained stimulation of β-cell by SU and increased oxidative stress.[8,15] Additionally findings that antioxidant treatment in animal models of T2DM protect β-cell damage further suggest that oxidative stress also has an important role to play in β-cell apoptosis. A study examining the dose dependent effects of different SU has shown that gliclazide did not significantly stimulate reactive oxygen species production.[15]

Beta-cell Dedifferentiation

Pancreatic β-cells respond to progression of T2DM by increasing production and secretion of insulin and also by increasing β-cell replication to overcome the insulin resistance. However, this adaptation is reversible, as evident from the fact that β-cell function returns after bariatric surgery in T2DM. But if the metabolic stress continues, β-cells succumb to the metabolic overload and dedifferentiation occurs. All together, these changes result in the escalation of the disease and eventually to a non-recoverable loss of a functionally mature β-cell mass.[16]

Beta-cell dedifferentiation may account for reduced β-cell mass and insulin secretion in patients with T2DM. An investigation conducted in early T2DM cases to assess the influence of exenatide, sitagliptin, and glimepiride on the secretory potential of β-cell revealed that glimepiride improved the secretion potential; however, exenatide or sitagliptin did not show such effects (functional β-cell mass). Present research data is not favorable with the proposal that SU have detrimental effects on β-cell mass or activity, especially the newer second-generation SU. In contrast, they seem to enhance secretory potential of β-cell if administered in the initial stages of T2DM.[17]

Weight Gain

Sulfonylureas are linked with weight gain which can be explained by their insulinotropic actions, reduction of glycosuria, and increased caloric intake to prevent/treat hypoglycemia. In the UKPDS, patients on SU monotherapy gained more weight compared to those on dietary intervention. However, second-generation SUs cause lesser weight gain as compared to first-generation SU as evident from the UKPDS study in which it was found that in the cohort at 10 years, patients who were assigned chlorpropamide gained 2.6 kg more ($p < 0.001$) while those assigned glibenclamide gained 1.7 kg more ($p < 0.001$) as compared to the conventional treatment.[18,19] Second-generation SUs such as glimepiride, glipizide XL, and gliclazide MR have established weight neutrality during the first year of therapy.[20-22] Several studies have suggested that once daily administration of glimepiride was associated with weight neutralizing or even reducing effect with weight loss up to 3 kg.[23] When compared to glibenclamide, glimepiride was associated with a significantly greater decrease in bodyweight/body mass index (-2.04 ± 3.99 kg vs. -0.58 ± 3.65 kg, $p < 0.001$; -0.71 ± 1.38 kg/m^2 vs. -0.20 ± 1.28 kg/m^2, $p < 0.001$, respectively) while providing equivalent glycemic control.[24] The ADVANCE trial after 5 years of follow-up showed no weight gain in T2DM patients treated with gliclazide MR.[25] In the GUIDE study, over the 27-week period of follow-up, body weight was stable with mean changes from 83.1 to 83.6 kg and 83.7 to 84.3 kg on gliclazide MR and glimepiride, respectively.[22] Choice of SU especially second-generation SU may be relevant in the context of overweight T2DM patients.[26]

Hypoglycemia

Jennings et al. reported that among the patients treated with SUs, up to 20% had symptoms suggestive of hypoglycemia, although in this study episodes were not always corroborated by plasma glucose determinations.[27] Hypoglycemia induced by SU treatment requiring assistance occurs in about 1 in every 100 persons per year.[28] A 10-year followup analysis of the UKPDS demonstrated that annual incidence of at least one hypoglycemic event was 17.7% with SU, almost half than those occurring with insulin, i.e., 36.5%.[18]

Individual SUs differ in their hypoglycemic potential owing to the differences in duration of action, time of administration, dose equivalence and potency of hypoglycemic action. Long-acting SUs such as glibenclamide are more likely to cause hypoglycemia.[26] Glimepiride is characterized by long duration of action; fewer hypoglycemic reactions as compared to glibenclamide (105 episodes vs. 150 episodes) were observed in a prospective double bind trial, possibly because of a better modulation of insulin release.[29] Gliclazide treated patients have been shown to experience lower rates of severe hypoglycemia in a recent systemic review and meta-analysis of clinical trials.[30] Previously, the GUIDE study demonstrated significantly lower rates of confirmed hypoglycemia [blood glucose (BG) <3 mmol/L] with gliclazide MR as compared to glimepiride (3.7% vs. 8.9%; $p = 0.003$). However, there were no episodes of hypoglycemia requiring external assistance in either arms.[22]

Careful phenotyping of the patient, a thorough assessment for all conditions which may result in SU induced hypoglycemia and precise choice of the agent is recommended.

Cardiovascular Safety

The UKPDS established that SUs do not cause macrovascular complications or mortality in T2DM.[18] This advantage continued for about a decade in those who had achieved optimal glycemic control. Identical outcomes had been revealed from 15 well-designed RCTs spanning over an extended period of 72 weeks. ADOPT, ADVANCE and ADVANCE-ON all of which showed no relation between SU therapy and a higher CV risk or mortality.[31-35]

Administration of current second-generation SU, namely, gliclazide MR and glimepiride in T2DM cases are related with reduced susceptibility of all-cause and CV-related mortality in contrast to regular or first-generation SU.[36-38] A latest case-control trial revealed that the possibility of occurrence of coronary artery disease (CAD) raised by 2.4 times ($p = 0.004$) with glibenclamide and twice ($p = 0.099$) with glipizide. On the other hand, the risk reduced by 0.3 times ($p = 0.385$) with glimepiride and 0.4 times ($p = 0.192$) with gliclazide.[39]

The results of the recent Cardiovascular Outcome Study of Linagliptin versus Glimepiride in Patients with Type 2 Diabetes (CAROLINA) demonstrated no difference in the composite of time to CV death, nonfatal myocardial infarction, or nonfatal stroke between the linagliptin and glimepiride groups.[40,41]

Ischemic Preconditioning

Glimepiride has been shown to preserve myocardial preconditioning with few CV adverse event in contrast to glibenclamide ($p = 0.01$ vs. $p = 0.34$, respectively).[42,43] The outcome of the latest national registry was identical; susceptibility to acute myocardial infarction was considerably lesser in second-generation SU (gliclazide MR, glimepiride) as against glibenclamide (2.7% vs. 7.5%; $p = 0.019$).[44] With these results, the favorable influence of second-generation SU in maintaining myocardial IPC has been established even though glibenclamide and glimepiride both show affinity toward SUR2 receptor.[5,42] In addition glimepiride has faster and extended period of action, in spite of reduced stimulation of insulin secretion as against glibenclamide.[45,46]

All-cause Mortality

Varying risk of nonfatal CV outcomes and all-cause mortality has been reported by recent retrospective SU studies, indicating the lack of class effect.[8] A meta-analysis evaluating all-cause mortality risk among SU reported the RR of death of different SUs versus glibenclamide to be: 0.65 (95% CI 0.53–0.79) for gliclazide, 0.83 (0.68–1.00) for glimepiride, 0.98 (0.80–1.19) for glipizide, 1.13 (0.90–1.42) for tolbutamide, and 1.34 (0.98–1.86) for chlorpropamide.[37] However, a retrospective study by Pantalone et al. found no significant difference in the overall mortality risk among individual SU (glyburide, glipizide, or glimepiride) in the entire cohort and concluded that choice of SU does not substantially influence over all mortality. However there was evidence of a trend that in those patients with documented CAD, the over-all mortality was reduced in patients taking glimepiride.[47]

A meta-analysis of 14 trials comparing SU versus metformin monotherapy found that SUs do not significantly affect all-cause mortality (RR 0.98; 95% CI 0.61–1.58) or CV mortality (RR 1.47; 95% CI 0.54–4.01) when compared to metformin in T2DM patients. However, SU decreased the risk of nonfatal macrovascular outcomes significantly (RR 0.67; 95% CI 0.48–0.93).[48] Similar results were observed in a Danish nationwide study which demonstrated no significant difference between gliclazide and metformin for all-cause mortality in both sets of patients, i.e., with and without previous myocardial infarction [hazard ratio (HR) 1.05; 95% CI 0.94–1.16 and 0.90 (0.68–1.20), respectively].[49] Studies evaluating the risk of all-cause mortality of metformin SU combination as compared to metformin insulin combination concluded that among patients with T2DM using metformin, the addition of insulin was associated with an increased risk of a composite of nonfatal CV outcomes and all-cause mortality as compared to addition of SU.[50]

PLACE OF SECOND-GENERATION SULFONYLUREAS IN CURRENT SCENARIO

For the treatment of T2DM, SUs still command an important position in guidelines across the world. Although concerns have been raised regarding safety of these drugs, the modern second-generation SU have been able to allay those fears to rest. In the light of the heterogeneous nature of T2DM, SUs are likely to continue to be a reliable and effective treatment, particularly as combination therapy. With insulin resistance and defects in insulin secretion being the main contributing factors for the development and progression of hyperglycemia, agents that can tackle these main pathogenic mechanisms represent a rational therapeutic approach. In T2DM patients with a predominant defect in insulin secretion, modern second-generation SUs can be a good choice as a frontline treatment. In addition second-generation SUs such as glimepiride, gliclazide, and glipizide are reliable and effective in glucose lowering and therefore continue to be an important option in the armamentarium for the treatment of T2DM.[7]

CONCLUSION

Second-generation SU continue to be an important option in the management of patients with T2DM owing to their well-established glycemic efficacy, safety, tolerability as well as cost-effectiveness. Considering the fact that many of the clinical concerns associated with the use of SU are agent specific and not class specific, a careful choice of specific SU should be considered for beneficial results. With better glycemic efficacy, long-term outcomes and low medication cost, once again, authors wish to emphasize that modern second generation SU remain as first line agents in the treatment of T2DM. Proper patient selection, choice of drug and dose, patient education and empowerment, and physician training will help ensure effective and safe use of this important class of drugs.

REFERENCES

1. Mogensen CE. Diabetes mellitus: a look at the past, a glimpse to the future. Medicographia. 2011;33:9-14.
2. Quianzon CC, Cheikh IE. History of current non-insulin medications for diabetes mellitus. J Community Hosp Intern Med Perspect. 2012;2:19081.
3. Blackburn H, Jacobs DR Jr. The University Group Diabetes Program 1961-1978: pioneering randomized controlled trial. Int J Epidemiol. 2017;46(5):1354–12.
4. Gerich JE. SU in the treatment of diabetes mellitus-1985. Mayo Clin Proc. 1985;60:439-43.
5. Basit A, Riaz M, Fawwad A. Glimepiride: evidence-based facts, trends, and observations (GIFTS). Vasc Health Risk Manag. 2012;8:463-72.

6. Jorgen R, Mia D, Lise G. History of the sulphonylureas. Diapedia. 2016;18: 8104336183.
7. Riddle MC. Modern SU: dangerous or wrongly accused? Diabetes Care. 2017;40:629-31.
8. Kalra S, Aamir AH, Raza A, Das AK, Khan AK, Shrestha D, et al. Place of SU in the management of type 2 diabetes mellitus in South Asia: A consensus statement. Indian J Endocr Metab. 2015;19:577-96.
9. King P, Peacock I, Donnelly R. The UK prospective diabetes study (UKPDS): clinical and therapeutic implications for type 2 diabetes: Therapeutic implications of the UKPDS. Br J Clin Pharmacol. 1999;48(5):643–8.
10. Heller SR, ADVANCE Collaborative Group. A summary of the ADVANCE trial. Diabetes Care. 2009;32(2):S357-5.
11. Wong MG, Perkovic V, Chalmers J, Woodward M, Li Q, Cooper ME et al. Long-term benefits of intensive glucose control for preventing end-stage kidney disease: ADVANCE-ON. Diabetes Care. 2016;39(5):694–7
12. Hayward RA, Reaven PD, Wiitala WL, Bahn GD, Reda DJ, Ge L et al. Follow-up of glycemic control and cardiovascular outcomes in type 2 diabetes. N Engl J Med. 2015;372(23):2197–10.
13. Thulé PM, Umpierrez G. SU: a new look at old therapy. Curr Diab Rep. 2014;14:473.
14. Maedler K, Carr RD, Bosco D, Zuellig RA, Berney T, Donath MY. Sulfonylurea induced beta-cell apoptosis in cultured human islets. J Clin Endocrinol Metab. 2005;90:501-6.
15. Sawada F, Inoguchi T, Tsubouchi H, Sasaki S, Fujii M, Maeda Y, et al. Differential effect of SU on production of reactive oxygen species and apoptosis in cultured pancreatic beta-cell line, MIN6. Metabolism. 2008;57:1038-45.
16. Blum B, Roose AN, Barrandon O, Maehr R, Arvanites AC, Davidow LS, et al. Reversal of β-cell de-differentiation by a small molecule inhibitor of the TGF β pathway. Elife. 2014;3:e02809.
17. Cinti F, Bouchi R, Kim-Muller JY, Ohmura Y, Sandoval PR, Masini M, et al. Evidence of β-Cell Dedifferentiation in Human Type 2 Diabetes. J Clin Endocrinol Metab. 2016;101:1044-54.
18. Turner R. Intensive blood glucose control with sulphonylureas or insulin compared with conventional treatment and risk of complications in patients with type 2 diabetes (UKPDS33). Lancet. 1998;352:837-53.
19. Olsson PO, Lindström T. Combination-therapy with bedtime NPH insulin and Sulphonylureas gives similar glycaemic control but lower weight gain than insulin twice daily in patients with type 2 diabetes. Diabetes Metab. 2002;28:272-7.
20. Bugos C, Austin M, Atherton T, Viereck C. Long term treatment of type 2 diabetes mellitus with glimepiride is weight neutral: a meta-analysis. Diabetes Res Clin Pract. 2000;50:S47.
21. Simonson DC, Kourides IA, Feinglos M, Shamoon H, Fischette CT. Efficacy, safety, and dose-response characteristics of glipizide gastrointestinal therapeutic system on glycemic control and insulin secretion in NIDDM. Results of two multicenter, randomized, placebo-controlled clinical trials. The Glipizide Gastrointestinal Therapeutic System Study Group. Diabetes Care. 1997;20:597-606.
22. Schernthaner G, Grimaldi A, Di Mario U, Drzewoski J, Kempler P, Kvapil M, et al. GUIDE study: Double blind comparison of once daily gliclazide MR and glimepiride in type 2 diabetic patients. Eur J Clin Invest. 2004;34: 535-42.
23. Hydrie MZ, Gul A, Hakeem R, Ahmadani MY, Basit A. Glimepiride study on type-2 diabetic subjects. Pak J Med Sci. 2006;22:132-5.
24. Martin S, Kolb H, Beuth J, van Leendert R, Schneider B, Scherbaum WA. Change in patients' body weight after 12 months of treatment with glimepiride or glibenclamide in type 2 diabetes: a multi centre retrospective cohort study. Diabetologia. 2003;46:1611-7.

25. Zoungas S, Chalmers J, Neal B, Billot L, Li Q, Hirakawa Y, et al. Follow up of blood pressure lowering and glucose control in type 2 diabetes. N Engl J Med. 2014;371:1392-406.
26. Del Prato S, Pulizzi N. The place of SU in the therapy for type 2 diabetes mellitus. Metabolism. 2006;55: S20-7.
27. Jennings AM, Wilson RM, Ward JD. Symptomatic hypoglycaemia in NIDDM patients treated with oral hypoglycaemic agents. Diabetes Care. 1989;12:203-8.
28. Leese GP, Wang J, Broomhall J, Kelly P, Marsden A, Morrison W, et al. Frequency of severe hypoglycemia requiring emergency treatment in type 1 and type 2 diabetes: a population-based study of health servicer source use. Diabetes Care. 2003;26:1176-80.
29. Draeger KE, Wernicke-Panten T, Lomp HJ, Schuler E, Rosskamp R. Long-term treatment of type 2 diabetic patients with the new oral antidiabetic agent glimepiride (Amaryl): a double-blind comparison with glibenclamide. Horm Metab Res. 1996;28:419-25.
30. Landman GW, deBock GH, van Hateren KJ, van Dijk PR, Groenier KH, Gans RO, et al. Safety and efficacy of gliclazide as treatment for type 2 diabetes: A systematic review and meta-analysis of randomized trials. PLoS One. 2014;9:e82880.
31. Feinglos MN, Bethel MA. Therapy of type 2 diabetes, cardiovascular death, and the UGDP. Am Heart J. 1999;138:S346-52.
32. Seltzer HS. A summary of criticisms of the findings and conclusions of the University Group Diabetes Program (UGDP). Diabetes. 1972;21:976-9.
33. Kilo C, Miller JP, Williamson JR. The Achilles heel of the University Group Diabetes Program. JAMA. 1980;243:450-7.
34. Holman RR, Paul SK, Bethel MA, Matthews DR, Neil HA. 10-year follow-up of intensive glucose control in type 2 diabetes. N Engl J Med. 2008;359:1577-89.
35. Rosenstock J, Marx N, Kahn SE, Zinman B, Kastelein JJ, Lachin JM, et al. Cardiovascular outcome trials in type 2 diabetes and the sulphonylurea controversy: Rationale for the active comparator CAROLINA trial. Diab Vasc Dis Res. 2013;10:289-301.
36. Selvin E, Bolen S, Yeh HC, Wiley C, Wilson LM, Marinopoulos SS, et al. Cardiovascular outcomes in trials of oral diabetes medications: a systematic review. Arch Intern Med. 2008;168:2070-80.
37. Simpson SH, Lee J, Choi S, Vandermeer B, Abdelmoneim AS, Featherstone TR. Mortality risk among SU: a systematic review and network meta-analysis. Lancet Diabetes Endocrinol. 2015;3:43-51.
38. Monami M, Genovese S, Mannucci E. Cardiovascular safety of SU: A meta-analysis of randomized clinical trials. Diabetes Obes Metab. 2013;15: 938-53.
39. Sadikot SM, Mogensen CE. Risk of coronary artery disease associated with initial sulphonylureas treatment of patients with type 2 diabetes: a matched case-control study. Diabetes Res Clin Pract. 2008;82:391-5.
40. Azoulay L, Suissa S. SU and the risks of cardiovascular events and death: a methodological meta-regression analysis of the observational studies. Diabetes Care. 2017;40:706-14.
41. Rosenstock J, Kahn SE, Johansen OE, Zinman B, Espeland MA, Woerle HJ, et al. Effect of Linagliptin vs Glimepiride on Major Adverse Cardiovascular Outcomes in Patients With Type 2 Diabetes: The CAROLINA Randomized Clinical Trial. JAMA. 2019;322(12):1155-66.
42. Mocanu MM, Maddock HL, Baxter GF, Lawrence CL, Standen NB, Yellon DM. Glimepiride, a novel Sulfonylurea, does not abolish myocardial protection afforded by either ischemic preconditioning or diazoxide. Circulation. 2001;103:3111-6.
43. Klepzig H, Kober G, Matter C, Luus H, Schneider H, Boedeker KH, et al. SU and ischaemic preconditioning; a double-blind, placebo-controlled evaluation of glimepiride and glibenclamide. Eur Heart J. 1999;20:439-46.

44. Zeller M, Danchin N, Simon D, Vahanian A, Lorgis L, Cottin Y, et al. Impact of type of preadmission SU on mortality and cardiovascular outcomes in diabetic patients with acute myocardial infarction. J Clin Endocrinol Metab. 2010;95:4993-5002.
45. Geisen K. Special pharmacology of the new Sulfonylurea glimepiride. Arzneimittelforschung. 1988;38:1120-30.
46. Kar P, Holt RI. The effect of sulphonylureas on the microvascular and macrovascular complications of diabetes. Cardiovasc Drugs Ther. 2008;22:207-13.
47. Pantalone KM, Kattan MW, Yu C, Wells BJ, Arrigain S, Jain A, et al. The risk of overall mortality in patients with type 2 diabetes receiving glipizide, glyburide, or glimepiride monotherapy: a retrospective analysis. Diabetes Care. 2010;33:1224-9.
48. Hemmingsen B, Schroll JB, Wetterslev J, Gluud C, Vaag A, Sonne DP, et al. Sulfonylurea versus metformin monotherapy in patients with type 2 diabetes: a Cochrane systematic review and meta-analysis of randomized clinical trials and trial sequential analysis. CMAJ Open. 2014;2:E162-75.
49. Schramm TK, Gislason GH, Vaag A, Rasmussen JN, Folke F, Hansen ML, et al. Mortality and cardiovascular risk associated with different insulin secretagogues compared with metformin in type 2 diabetes, with or without a previous myocardial infarction: a nationwide study. Eur Heart J. 2011;32:1900-8.
50. Roumie CL, Greevy RA, Grijalva CG, Hung AM, Liu X, Murff HJ, et al. Association between intensification of metformin treatment with insulin vs SU and cardiovascular events and all-cause mortality among patients with diabetes. JAMA. 2014;311:2288-96.

3

CHAPTER

Insulin Secretagogs: Nonsulfonylureas Glinides (Repaglinide and Nateglinide)

Rajeev Chawla, Shalini Jaggi

INTRODUCTION

The etiopathogenesis of type 2 diabetes mellitus (T2DM) that earlier implicated only an insulin secretory defect due to impaired β-cell function and increasing insulin resistance at the liver and muscle has evolved over time to the famous "ominous octet" proposal put forth by DeFronzo and now to the "dirty dozen" highlighting the contribution of delayed incretin response from the gut, increased glucagon secretion from the α-cells, the insulin resistance in the brain as well as increased glucose reabsorption in the kidneys, and deficiency of vitamin D, etc. in worsening hyperglycemia of diabetes. In most T2DM individuals, it is not just one but a multitude of these defects that need to be addressed together to achieve euglycemia, thus warranting the need for an individualized pathophysiology-based treatment strategy. The universal finding of progressive islet cell dysfunction on a background of insulin resistance still remains a core defect in all T2DM patients, characterized by the absence of first phase of insulin secretion that starts very early in the pathogenesis of hyperglycemia and eventually progresses with increasing decline in insulin secretion with time. The advent of novel therapies aimed at targeting different pathophysiological defects has opened wider avenues for a comprehensive diabetes management that can be tailor-made for each patient.

Drugs classified as insulin secretagogs address the core defect of declining insulin secretion and work by stimulating the pancreatic β-cells to augment insulin secretion—both first phase (release of preformed insulin) as well as second phase (conversion of proinsulin to insulin). For many years, sulfonylureas were the only class of secretagogs available, but even the most rapid acting of these was a little slow in restoring the very early insulin release immediately on feeding. The relatively newer agents, meglitinides, also called the nonsulfonylurea secretagogs have emerged as very effective agents, especially for managing postprandial hyperglycemia by augmenting early insulin response to meals.

Currently, two molecules (agents) of this drug class (Meglitinides) are available in the market—(1) repaglinide and (2) nateglinide. We provide a critical review of these novel nonsulfonylurea agents in our armamentarium against diabetes.

MEGLITINIDES

As mentioned above, these agents work in a manner slightly different from sulfonylureas.[1] Most importantly, they bind to the sulfonylurea receptor in the insulin producing β cells at a site that is different from the sulfonylurea-binding site (**Fig. 3.1**). Also, their interaction with the receptor is not as "tight" as that of sulfonylureas, resulting in not only a weaker affinity but also a faster dissociation clinically seen as a much shorter duration of action and a need for much higher blood glucose level to stimulate insulin secretion from the pancreas[2] thus making them very effective in controlling postmeal hyperglycemia.

Currently, the two available meglitinide molecules, namely nateglinide and repaglinide, are approved for use alone or in combination with all other diabetes agents (except offcourse sulfonylureas) in people with T2DM. The primary effect of these medications is the reduction of postmeal blood glucose levels, translating into an overall reduction in glycated hemoglobin levels.[3]

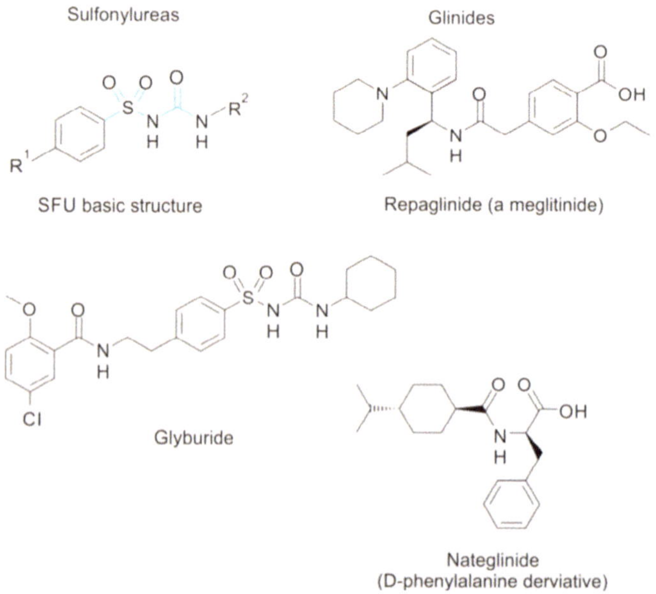

FIG. 3.1: Molecular structure of sulfonylureas and meglitinides.

Both these agents have relatively short half-lives (i.e., quickly disappear from the body) and should be taken 1–30 minutes before each major meal.

Repaglinide

Mechanism of Action

The blood glucose-lowering action of repaglinide involves a glucose-dependent stimulation of insulin release from the pancreatic β cells.[4] It causes closure of the adenosine triphosphate (ATP)-dependent potassium channels by binding to typical sites, other than the sulfonylurea (SU)-binding sites. This potassium channel closure causes depolarization of the β-cell membrane, which in turn opens the calcium channels resulting in influx of calcium ions. This calcium influx inside the β cell stimulates release of insulin resulting in stimulation of insulin secretion. This ion channel action is highly tissue-specific in the β cells, with very low affinity for channels in the heart and skeletal muscle (**Fig. 3.2**).

Indications and Usage

Repaglinide is indicated for use in adults with T2DM as an adjunct to diet and exercise to improve glycemic control.

Contraindications

The United States Food and Drug Administration (USFDA) prohibits use of repaglinide in patients with:

- Type 1 diabetes mellitus (T1DM)
- Diabetic ketoacidosis, with or without coma, where insulin is the only recommended agent for use

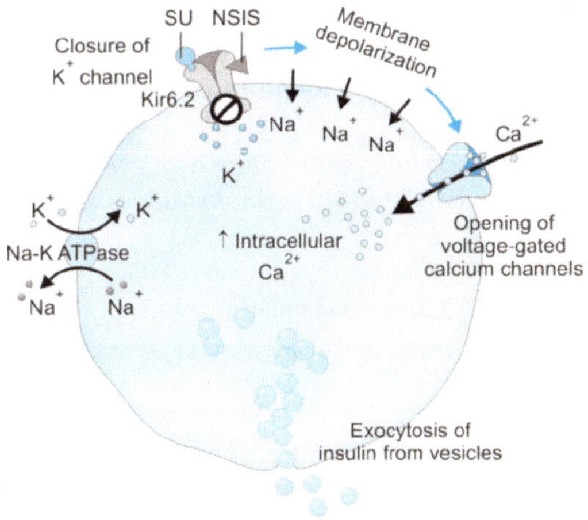

(SU: sulfonylurea; NSIS: nonsulfonylurea insulin secretagogs; Na: sodium; K: potassium; Ca: calcium; Na-K ATPase: sodium potassium adenosine triphosphatase)

FIG. 3.2: Mechanism of action of insulin secretagogs.

- Coadministration of gemfibrozil
- Known hypersensitivity to the drug or its inactive ingredients.

Dosing (Adults)

Route of administration: Oral

Time of administration: Repaglinide can be taken immediately before a meal up to maximum 30 minutes prior to the meal, though ideally 15 minutes prior to a meal is the most common time recommended.

Starting dose: It can be started with 0.5 mg up to thrice a day before each meal for drug-naïve patients with a glycated hemoglobin (HbA1c) below 8.0%. For all others, the recommended starting dose is 1–2 mg taken up to three times daily, prior to each main meal. Uptitrate after 1–2 weeks if no response to maximum 4 mg per meal to a maximum recommended daily dose of 16 mg/day (i.e., 4 mg prior to each meal four times daily) although 2 mg three times a day is usually an optimum dose.

The drug can be used as monotherapy or combined with all other agents recommended for T2DM management, except sulfonylureas. Dose adjustments can be made depending on the blood glucose levels to avoid hypoglycemia and attain target HbA1c levels individualized for the patient. If suitable drug combination therapies fail to achieve the target levels, consider discontinuing therapy and starting insulin as per the recommendations.

Drug–drug Interactions

Repaglinide interacts with certain other drugs, particularly gemfibrozil as well as combination of gemfibrozil and itraconazole, which raise blood levels of repaglinide roughly 28- to 72-fold, respectively.

Dose adjustments are necessary in people with severe kidney dysfunction and moderate-to-severe liver dysfunction (**Table 3.1**).

Repaglinide is shown to cause more hypoglycemia as well as weight gain than nateglinide in various studies.

TABLE 3.1: **Dosing adjustment in renal impairment.**

Renal impairment	Drug dose
Creatinine clearance (CrCl) 40–80 mL/min (mild-to-moderate renal dysfunction)	Initial dosage adjustment does not appear to be necessary
CrCl 20–40 mL/min	Initiate 0.5 mg with meals; titrate carefully
<20 mL/min or hemodialysis	No studies conducted

Nateglinide

Mechanism of Action

The mechanism of action of nateglinide is same as repaglinide, i.e., stimulation of insulin release from the β cells in the pancreatic islets,[4] which diminishes at lower glucose levels. It closes ATP-dependent potassium channels on the β-cell membrane by binding to non-SU sites, which depolarizes the β-cell membrane and opens calcium channels. The consequent calcium influx induces insulin secretion in a glucose-dependent manner. Nateglinide has a high tissue selectivity and a low affinity for the skeletal muscle.

Indications and Usage

Nateglinide is indicated as an adjunct to diet and exercise to improve glycemic control in adults with T2DM.

Contraindications

Nateglinide is contraindicated in patients with:
- Type 1 diabetes mellitus
- Diabetic ketoacidosis
- Known hypersensitivity to the drug or its inactive ingredients.

Dosing (Adults)

Recommended dose is 120 mg three times a day prior to each major meal, though it may be initiated at 60 mg three times a day and uptitrated to achieve desired glycemic control over 1–2 weeks.

Route of administration: Oral

Time of administration: Ideally 15 minutes before a major meal, but may vary from immediately before a meal to maximum 30 minutes prior to the meal. In case a meal is skipped, the scheduled dose should be omitted to reduce hypoglycemia risk.

Safe for use in elderly age group, however, caution is advised to rule out hypoglycemia.

Dose adjustment in hepatic impairment:
- Mild hepatic insufficiency—Increased serum levels seen. No dose adjustment needed.
- Moderate-to-severe hepatic insufficiency—Not studied. Use with caution (**Table 3.2**).

Since these agents are also insulin secretagogs working like sulfonylureas, they also carry a risk of hypoglycemia. However, this risk is much lower as compared with sulfonylureas and this can be attributed to their glucose-dependent action and a shorter half-life.[5,6] Weight gain with these agents is also somewhat less when compared with sulfonylureas. These compounds are metabolized in the liver through the cytochrome P450 system and hence are contraindicated in patients with severe liver

TABLE 3.2: Pharmacological profile of meglitinides.

Drugs	Action of duration (hours)	Dose range (mg)	Number of doses	Common adverse effects
Repaglinide	2–6	0.5, 1, and 2	Two to four	Hypoglycemia, headache, and weight gain
Nateglinide	1–3	180–360	Two to four	Hypoglycemia, diarrhea, and dizziness

dysfunction; the dose should also be reduced in those with severe renal dysfunction. Nausea, diarrhea, dizziness, and lightheadedness are the most common adverse effects seen with this class of agents.

Due to shorter half-life and short duration of action, these agents stimulate insulin release briefly and in a glucose-dependent manner. The insulin concentration increase is dose dependent with an incremental peak occurring about 2 hours after drug administration. In view of their pharmacological properties, these agents are best administered just prior to major meals as they help control the prandial glycemic surges. These drugs can be timed with major meals and are considered a suitable option for those patients who follow flexible meal timings and in the elderly. Patients are advised to skip a dose if the meal is missed. Out of the two agents in this class, repaglinide is as effective as metformin or sulfonylureas in terms of glycemic control while nateglinide is somewhat less potent.

Numerous trials and meta-analysis have validated various therapies for T2DM after balancing their actions and benefits with their side effect profiles.[7] However, despite our best efforts, we are still far from where we can not only effectively treat the diabetic patients but also reverse the diabetes process. An early diagnosis when the metabolic abnormalities are usually less severe and an appropriate use of pathophysiology-based pharmacotherapy can be rewarding in reducing the burden of diabetes complications. Repaglinide and nateglinide are two nonsulfonylurea insulin secretagogs binding to the sulfonylurea receptor at a site different from the sulfonylurea-binding site, thus working as oral hypoglycemic agents that help in achieving a modest HbA1c reduction with much less hypoglycemia than the more potent sulfonylureas, creating their niche place among secretagogs in the management of T2DM.

CONCLUSION

Type 2 diabetes mellitus is characterised by various pathophysiological defects and targeting these multiple mechanisms forms the basis of an individualised management approach. Meglitinides have fast gained popularity as potent oral hypoglycemic agents owing to their mechanism of action through potentiation of insulin secretion by binding to sites other than the SU-binding sites on the ATP dependent potassium channels on the beta cell membrane. Their shorter half life and shorter duration of action makes them preferred agents in controlling postprandial hyperglycemia especially due to much lesser potential for causing hypoglycemia than the more potent and longer acting sulfonylureas. Both nateglinide and repaglinide have been found to be safe, even in the elderly population and can be prescribed especially in patients following flexible meal timings, without a major concern of hypoglycemia. Hence these nonsulfonylurea secretagogs find a place of preference amongst other agents where both efficacy and less propensity for hypoglycemia are the important deciding factors determining the choice of agent in the T2DM management treatment strategies.

REFERENCES

1. Dunning BE. New non-sulfonylurea insulin secretagogues Expert Opin Investig Drugs. 1997;6(8):1041-8.
2. Marino M. (2009). Diabetes self-management: Meglitinides. [online] Available from https://www.diabetesselfmanagement.com/blog/meglitinides/. [Last accessed February, 2020].
3. Perfetti R, Ahmad A. Novel sulfonylurea and non-sulfonylurea drugs to promote the secretion of insulin. Trends Endocrinol Metab. 2000;11(6):218-23.
4. DailyMed. (2019). DailyMed Database. [online] Available from https://dailymed.nlm.nih.gov/dailymed/. [Last accessed February, 2020].
5. Inzucchi SE, Bergenstal RM, Buse JB, Diamant M, Ferrannini E, Nauck M, et al. Management of hyperglycemia in type 2 diabetes: a patient-centered approach. Position statement of the American Diabetes Association (ADA) and the European Association for the Study of Diabetes (EASD). Diabetes Care. 2012;35(6):1364-79.
6. Management of type 2 diabetes: consensus of diabetes organizations Elaena Quattrocchi, BS, PharmD, FASHP, CDE,corresponding author Tamara Goldberg, BS, PharmD, BCPS, and Nino Marzella, BS, MS, PharmD Drugs Context. 2020; 9: 212607. Published online 2020 Jan 27. doi: 10.7573/dic.212607
7. Cheng AYY, Fantus IG. Oral antihyperglycemic therapy for type 2 diabetes mellitus. CMAJ. 2005;172(2):213-26.

4

CHAPTER

Metformin

Vishnu Vardhan Garla

INTRODUCTION

Metformin is the recommended initial glucose-lowering agent for the treatment of type 2 diabetes mellitus (T2DM). It is one of the most commonly prescribed medications and is listed as an essential medication in the World Health Organization (WHO) model list of essential medications. Metformin is also being investigated for use in polycystic ovary syndrome (PCOS), cancer prevention, and as an antiaging agent.

HISTORY

Galega officinalis, a herb rich in guanidine, was used to treat symptoms of diabetes mellitus (DM) (increased thirst and urination) as early as 1772. In the 1930s, guanidine derivatives were first used to treat DM but soon fell out of favor with the discovery and availability of insulin.[1] In the 1940s, metformin was studied as a potential antimalarial drug.[2] Jean Sterne was the first to use metformin to treat diabetes in 1957.[3] Initially, its role in the treatment of DM was limited as more potent biguanides (phenformin and buformin) were available. However, phenformin was discontinued in the 1970s due to the high risk of lactic acidosis. Metformin was introduced to the USA in 1995 and added to the WHO list of essential medications in 2011.[4]

MECHANISM OF ACTION

Metformin is the first-line medication for the treatment of T2DM and also has potential antitumor and antiaging effects; however, the molecular pathways through which it acts are yet to be elucidated. Around 70% of metformin dose is absorbed in the small intestine and the rest is eliminated in the feces. After absorption, metformin is concentrated in the liver, intestines, kidneys, and bladder. The peak concentration after an oral dose occurs in 2 hours and the half-life is 4–5 hours. Metformin does not bind to plasma proteins and is eliminated unchanged in the urine.[5]

Metformin predominantly acts on the liver by inhibiting hepatic gluconeogenesis. It is taken up by the hepatocytes via organic cation transporter 1 (OCT1) and inhibits complex I of the respiratory chain, decreasing adenosine triphosphate (ATP) production. The decrease in ATP production activates adenosine monophosphate protein kinase (AMPK), which activates process increasing ATP production and inhibits those consuming ATP. Metformin can also activate AMPK via a lysosomal pathway involving AXIN and mammalian target of rapamycin (mTOR).[5]

Recently, there has been an increase in attention to the effect of metformin on the gut as its antihyperglycemic effect cannot be explained entirely by its hepatic action.[6] Even in patients with mutations in *SLC22A1* (the gene encoding OCT1) leading to reduced uptake of metformin in the liver, its ability to reduce glucose remains intact.[7] Metformin increases anaerobic glucose metabolism in the enterocytes, as evidenced by increased intestinal fluorodeoxyglucose (FDG) uptake on positron emission tomography (PET) scans.[8] There is also a concurrent increase in AMPK metabolism in colonic enterocytes, which suggests increased glucose metabolism. Other potential mechanisms involving the gut are increasing the secretion of glucagon-like peptide-1 (GLP-1), suppression of hepatic glucose production through action via nucleus tractus solitarius, and alteration of the intestinal microbiome (**Fig. 4.1**).[9]

EFFECT ON GUT MICROBIOME

The role of gut microbiota in the pathogenesis of DM and obesity has been recently recognized. Metagenomic studies have revealed lower levels of butyrate-producing bacteria in patients with T2DM.[10] These metabolites can affect insulin resistance. Biguanides have been known to have antimicrobial activity and have been used as antimalarials in the past.[1] The concentration of metformin in the gut can be up to 100-fold as in the blood. Besides the concentration of the drug, transit time and rate of absorption determine the level of exposure explaining the variability of the gut action of metformin. Metformin has been shown to increase the abundance of short-chain fatty acid-producing bacteria, increasing the ability to produce butyrate and propionate, which in turn could decrease insulin resistance.[11]

TREATMENT OF TYPE 2 DIABETES MELLITUS

Metformin is the first-line treatment for T2DM to achieve glycemic targets. Garber et al. showed that the effect of metformin

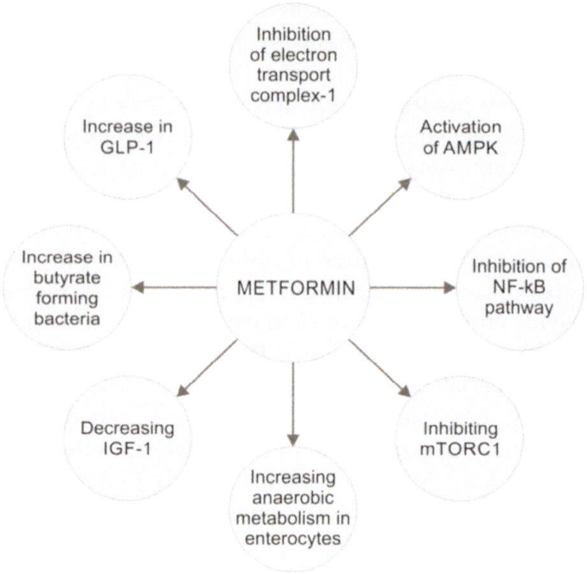

(AMPK: adenosine monophosphate protein kinase; GLP-1: glucagon-like peptide-1; IGF-1: insulin-like growth factor-1; NF-kB: nuclear factor-kappa B; mTORC1: mammalian target of rapamycin)

FIG. 4.1: The multifaceted action of metformin.

was dose dependent, with the minimal effective dose being 500 mg daily and the maximal dose was 2,000 mg daily. Metformin reduces glycated hemoglobin (HbA1c) by 1–1.5%. Metformin is also useful when used in combination with other antihyperglycemic agents due to its unique action and lack of hypoglycemic potential.[12]

DIABETES PREVENTION

The impact that a diagnosis of DM has both on the patient and the healthcare system is enormous; therefore, prevention of the same is of essential importance. Metformin is considered a potential agent in the prevention of DM due to its mechanism of action, favorable side effect profile, and ease of accessibility.[13] DPPOS (Diabetes Prevention Program Outcomes Study) evaluated the role of metformin in preventing the onset of DM in high-risk participants. The DPP study showed that at the end of 5 years, there was a 31% decrease in the incidence of DM with the use of metformin as compared to placebo.[14] Similarly, the DPPOS study showed an 18% decrease in the onset of DM at 15 years with metformin use.[15,16] Around 64% of metformin's efficacy in preventing DM were attributed to its ability to cause weight loss.[17] Younger participants, women with a history of gestational diabetes mellitus (GDM), those with a body mass index (BMI) >35 kg/m^2, or higher fasting blood sugars were likely to benefit the most with metformin use.[14,18]

PREGNANCY AND GESTATIONAL DIABETES MELLITUS

Traditionally, metformin therapy has always been stopped in pregnancy. Metformin crosses the placenta and attains a similar concentration in the fetal blood as maternal blood.[19] However, animal studies have shown no increase in congenital malformations or miscarriages. Cassina et al. studied 351 women with PCOS and found no increase in congenital anomalies or miscarriages with metformin exposure in early pregnancy.[20] Rowan et al., in the metformin in gestational (MiG) DM study, showed no difference in outcomes between insulin and metformin. The offspring follow-up (TOFU) study showed no difference in total fat mass and incidence of hypertension in those exposed to either metformin or insulin in pregnancy.[21,22] Women with lower BMI and lower baseline glucose levels are more responsive and potential candidates for metformin monotherapy in GDM. In conclusion, metformin appears to be a safe option for the treatment of GDM; however, evidence from randomized trials is awaited and is presently not approved by the FDA for this indication.[23]

NONDIABETES MELLITUS USES

- *Antitumor effects*: The antitumor effects of metformin were first reported in hamsters in 2001.[24] Metformin's ability to inhibit the mTORC1, a potent growth promoter, is largely responsible for its antitumor effects. Metformin inhibits the passage of RagA-RaCGTase through the nuclear pore complex deactivating mTORC1 and inducing acyl-CoA dehydrogenase family member-10 (ACAD-10) which has been shown to increase life span. Metformin also decreases hyperinsulinemia and levels of insulin-like growth factor-1 (IGF-1), both of which are growth promoters. Lastly, metformin-induced decrease in glucose levels could potentially starve cancer cells of energy and decrease proliferation.[25]

  Various preclinical and epidemiological studies have shown metformin's efficacy in reducing the incidence of colorectal, ovarian, breast, and prostate cancer.[26-28] Furthermore, metformin has also been shown to increase cancer survival as well. However, these results have not been consistent. Multiple clinical trials appear promising with metformin successfully altering surrogate markers for various cancers; however, results from phase III studies are awaited.[29]
- *Antiaging*: Aging is a "deterioration in the maintenance of the homeostatic process over time, leading to an increased risk for disease and death".[30] An important mechanism of aging

is DNA damage by free radicals leading to ineffective protein translation. Metformin suppresses nuclear factor-kappa B (NF-kB) by activation of AMPK inhibiting the inflammatory response. It also decreases the production of reactive oxygen species and superoxide anions through inhibition of mTOR.[31] Metformin can also prevent the accumulation of ceramides in muscle, preventing myoblast senescence.[32] Clinically in small studies, metformin has been shown to decrease the risk of cardiovascular disease, dementia and improve depression, muscle strength, and mobility; however, evidence from large trials [TAME (Targeting Aging with Metformin), ePREDICE (Early Prevention of Diabetes Complications in People with Hyperglycemia in Europe), etc.] is awaited.[31]

- *Polycystic ovarian syndrome*: PCOS is a syndrome characterized by menstrual irregularities, clinical or biochemical hyperandrogenism, and the presence of multiple cysts on the ovaries. Metformin is commonly prescribed for the treatment of PCOS although it is not yet approved by the FDA for this indication. Hyperinsulinemia is a cardinal feature of PCOS secondary to impaired insulin-independent glucose disposal (IIGD). Metformin increases insulin sensitivity and resolves the hyperinsulinemia.[33] Although it lowers testosterone levels by 20–25%, it is not associated with clinically significant improvements in menstrual irregularities or hirsutism. Metformin does not improve clinical pregnancy or live birth rates in a significant manner. At present, metformin is indicated for the treatment of glucose intolerance/DM in women with PCOS.[34]

CONTRAINDICATIONS

Metformin is contraindicated in patients with known hypersensitivity to metformin, renal failure with a glomerular filtration rate (GFR) of <30 mL/min/1.73 m^2, and decompensated hepatic or heart failure.[35,36]

ADVERSE EFFECTS

- *Gastrointestinal side effects*: Gastrointestinal side effects with metformin include nausea, vomiting, abdominal pain, flatulence, and diarrhea. These side effects occur in 30% of metformin users; however, they are severe enough to warrant discontinuation in only about 5%. Various theories have been put forth to explain the occurrence of gastrointestinal side effects; these include an increase in lactate production by the enterocytes, alteration of the intestinal microbiome, and heterogeneity in OCT1 channel.

Initiating metformin at a low dose and slow upward titration and administration with meals may help decrease the occurrence of gastrointestinal (GI) side effects. Sustained-release metformin is associated with a lower occurrence and discontinuation rates from GI side effects. It is a viable option for patients who cannot tolerate immediate-release metformin.[37]

- *Lactic acidosis*: Metformin's association with lactic acidosis stems from historical data on phenformin, an older biguanide which had a well-known association with lactic acidosis. However, both these agents are pharmacologically different and lactic acidosis with metformin is extremely rare (0–0.09 per 100 patient-years). Metformin inhibits hepatic gluconeogenesis through inhibition of glycerophosphate dehydrogenase leading to decreased conversion of lactate to glucose. However, lactic acidosis rarely occurs due to an efficient Cori cycle, which clears the lactate from the liver. Metformin-induced lactic acidosis (MILA) can be seen in cases of metformin overdose with or without renal failure. The diagnosis requires a high level of lactate, acidosis, and high plasma concentration of metformin. Metformin-associated lactic acidosis (MALA) can occur when there is an increased production of lactate (respiratory or circulatory failure) or decreased clearance (liver failure) concurrent with metformin use. However, in these scenarios, metformin may be a silent bystander rather than an active contributor. It is challenging to distinguish MILA from MALA in clinical practice. Close monitoring of renal function and avoidance/discontinuation of metformin in patients with decompensated hepatic failure, unstable congestive heart failure, and alcohol abuse are recommended.[38]
- *Vitamin B12 deficiency*: Metformin has been associated with vitamin B12 deficiency. Regular monitoring and supplementation are recommended in patients on metformin therapy.[39]

FUTURE DIRECTIONS

Despite the widespread use of metformin, much remains to be known about it. Metformin is the first-line agent for the treatment of T2DM and is also increasingly used for the management of nondiabetic conditions. While it is promising, there is a necessity to obtain high-quality evidence to strengthen the role of metformin in reducing cardiovascular risk and preventing diabetes. Metformin's role in preventing cancer recurrence, antiaging, and reproductive health also needs confirmation with large scale studies. Further avenues of research include studying the role of metformin in altering gut microbiota.

REFERENCES

1. Bailey CJ. Metformin: historical overview. Diabetologia. 2017;60(9):1566-76.
2. Curd FHS, Davey DG, Rose FL. Studies on synthetic antimalarial drugs; Some biguanide derivatives as new types of antimalarial substances with both therapeutic and causal prophylactic activity. Ann Trop Med Parasitol. 1945;39:208-16.
3. Sterne J. Du nouveau dans les antidiabétiques. La NN dimethylamine guanyl guanidine (N.N.D.G.). Maroc Med. 1957;36:1295-6.
4. DeFronzo RA, Goodman AM. Efficacy of metformin in patients with non-insulin-dependent diabetes mellitus. The Multicenter Metformin Study Group. N Engl J Med. 1995;333(9):541-9.
5. Rena G, Hardie DG, Pearson ER. The mechanisms of action of metformin. Diabetologia. 2017;60(9):1577-85.
6. Bailey CJ, Wilcock C, Scarpello JH. Metformin and the intestine. Diabetologia. 2008;51(8):1552-3.
7. Sundelin E, Gormsen LC, Jensen JB, Vendelbo MH, Jakobsen S, Munk OL, et al. Genetic Polymorphisms in Organic Cation Transporter 1 Attenuates Hepatic Metformin Exposure in Humans. Clin Pharmacol Ther. 2017;102(5):841-8.
8. Massollo M, Marini C, Brignone M, Emionite L, Salani B, Riondato M, et al. Metformin temporal and localized effects on gut glucose metabolism assessed using 18F-FDG PET in mice. J Nucl Med. 2013;54(2):259-66.
9. DeFronzo RA, Buse JB, Kim T, Burns C, Skare S, Baron A, et al. Once-daily delayed-release metformin lowers plasma glucose and enhances fasting and postprandial GLP-1 and PYY: results from two randomised trials. Diabetologia. 2016;59(8):1645-54.
10. Tilg H, Moschen AR. Microbiota and diabetes: an evolving relationship. Gut. 2014;63(9):1513-21.
11. Vallianou NG, Stratigou T, Tsagarakis S. Metformin and gut microbiota: their interactions and their impact on diabetes. Hormones (Athens). 2019;18(2): 141-4.
12. Sanchez-Rangel E, Inzucchi SE. Metformin: clinical use in type 2 diabetes. Diabetologia. 2017;60(9):1586-93.
13. Aroda VR, Knowler WC, Crandall JP, Perreault L, Edelstein SL, Jeffries SL, et al. Metformin for diabetes prevention: insights gained from the Diabetes Prevention Program/Diabetes Prevention Program Outcomes Study. Diabetologia. 2017;60(9):1601-11.
14. Knowler WC, Barrett-Connor E, Fowler SE, Hamman RF, Lachin JM, Walker EA, et al. Reduction in the incidence of type 2 diabetes with lifestyle intervention or metformin. N Engl J Med. 2002;346(6):393-403.
15. Diabetes Prevention Program Research Group, Knowler WC, Fowler SE, Hamman RF, Christophi CA, Hoffman HJ, et al. 10-year follow-up of diabetes incidence and weight loss in the Diabetes Prevention Program Outcomes Study. Lancet. 2009;374(9702):1677-86.
16. Diabetes Prevention Program Research Group. Long-term effects of lifestyle intervention or metformin on diabetes development and microvascular complications over 15-year follow-up: the Diabetes Prevention Program Outcomes Study. Lancet Diabetes Endocrinol. 2015;3(11):866-75.
17. Lachin JM, Christophi CA, Edelstein SL, Ehrmann DA, Hamman RF, Kahn SE, et al. Factors associated with diabetes onset during metformin versus placebo therapy in the Diabetes Prevention Program. Diabetes. 2007;56(4):1153-9.
18. Ratner RE, Christophi CA, Metzger BE, Dabelea D, Bennett PH, Pi-Sunyer X, et al. Prevention of diabetes in women with a history of gestational diabetes: Effects of metformin and lifestyle interventions. J Clin Endocrinol Metab. 2008;93(12):4774-9.
19. Charles B, Norris R, Xiao X, Hague W. Population pharmacokinetics of metformin in late pregnancy. Ther Drug Monit. 2006;28(1):67-72.

20. Cassina M, Donà M, Di Gianantonio E, Litta P, Clementi M. First-trimester exposure to metformin and risk of birth defects: a systematic review and meta-analysis. Hum Reprod Update. 2014;20(5):656-69.
21. Rowan JA, Hague WM, Gao W, Battin MR, Moore MP, MiG Trial Investigators. Metformin versus insulin for the treatment of gestational diabetes. N Engl J Med. 2008;358(19):2003-15.
22. Rowan JA, Rush EC, Obolonkin V, Battin M, Wouldes T, Hague WM. Metformin in gestational diabetes: the offspring follow-up (MiG TOFU): body composition at 2 years of age. Diabetes Care. 2011;34(10):2279-84.
23. DiaLindsay RS, Loeken MR. Metformin use in pregnancy: promises and uncertainties. Diabetologia. 2017;60(9):1612-9.
24. Schneider MB, Matsuzaki H, Haorah J, Ulrich A, Standop J, Ding XZ, et al. Prevention of pancreatic cancer induction in hamsters by metformin. Gastroenterology. 2001;120(5):1263-70.
25. Wang YW, He SJ, Feng X, Cheng J, Luo YT, Tian L, et al. Metformin: a review of its potential indications. Drug Des Devel Ther. 2017;11:2421-9.
26. Tseng CH. Metformin reduces ovarian cancer risk in Taiwanese women with type 2 diabetes mellitus. Diabetes Metab Res Rev. 2015;31(6):619-26.
27. Jiralerspong S, Palla SL, Giordano SH, Meric-Bernstam F, Liedtke C, Barnett CM, et al. Metformin and pathologic complete responses to neoadjuvant chemotherapy in diabetic patients with breast cancer. J Clin Oncol. 2009; 27(20):3297-302.
28. Tseng CH. Metformin significantly reduces incident prostate cancer risk in Taiwanese men with type 2 diabetes mellitus. Eur J Cancer. 2014;50(16): 2831-7.
29. Heckman-Stoddard BM, DeCensi A, Sahasrabuddhe VV, Ford LG. Repurposing metformin for the prevention of cancer and cancer recurrence. Diabetologia. 2017;60(9):1639-47.
30. Losordo DW, Henry TD. New definition of aging? Measuring regenerative capacity in patients. Circ Res. 2016;119(7):774-5.
31. Valencia WM, Palacio A, Tamariz L, Florez H. Metformin and ageing: improving ageing outcomes beyond glycaemic control. Diabetologia. 2017;60(9):1630-8.
32. Jadhav KS, Dungan CM, Williamson DL. Metformin limits ceramide-induced senescence in C2C12 myoblasts. Mech Ageing Dev. 2013;134(11-12):548-59.
33. Sam S, Ehrmann DA. Metformin therapy for the reproductive and metabolic consequences of polycystic ovary syndrome. Diabetologia. 2017;60(9):1656-61.
34. McCartney CR, Marshall JC. Clinical Practice. Polycystic Ovary Syndrome. N Engl J Med. 2016;375(1):54-64.
35. Garla V, Yanes-Cardozo L, Lien LF. Current therapeutic approaches in the management of hyperglycemia in chronic renal disease. Rev Endocr Metab Disord. 2017;18(1):5-19.
36. Glucophage®. Glucophage® XR (metformin hydrochloride) Extended-release Tablets. New York: Bristol-Myers Squibb Company; 2017.
37. Bonnet F, Scheen A. Understanding and overcoming metformin gastrointestinal intolerance. Diabetes Obes Metab. 2017;19(4):473-81.
38. Salvatore T, Pafundi PC, Marfella R, Sardu C, Rinaldi L, Monaco L, et al. Metformin lactic acidosis: Should we still be afraid? Diabetes Res Clin Pract. 2019;157:107879.
39. Chapman LE, Darling AL, Brown JE. Association between metformin and vitamin B(12) deficiency in patients with type 2 diabetes: A systematic review and meta-analysis. Diabetes Metab. 2016;42(5):316-27.

5

CHAPTER

Incretin-based Therapies: Dipeptidyl Peptidase-4 Inhibitors

Chaitanya K Mamillapalli

INTRODUCTION

Glucagon-like peptide-1 (GLP-1) is synthesized by L cells (found in ileum and colon) and glucose-dependent insulinotropic polypeptide (GIP) is produced by K cells (found in duodenum).[1] These peptides have a high degree of homology that are termed as incretins and are secreted in response to eating a meal. Oral glucose results in a greater secretion of plasma insulin concentrations than intravenous glucose infusion and this phenomenon is termed as incretin effect. In healthy individuals, up to 60% of insulin release in the postprandial phase is due to the incretin effect. After absorption into the hepatic portal circulation, GLP-1 binds to GLP-1 receptors on pancreatic α and β cells. GLP-1 by its action on β cells makes pancreatic islets more sensitive to intracellular glucose level, enhancing the production of insulin in response to high blood glucose and by binding to α cells causes negative feedback on postmeal glucagon secretion. In addition, GLP-1 also slows gastric emptying. GIP promotes insulin secretion, but has no effect on glucagon secretion or gastric emptying.

Glucose-dependent insulinotropic polypeptide (GIP) and GLP-1 are rapidly degraded by the enzyme dipeptidyl peptidase-4 (DPP-4) and consequently have very short plasma half-lives (<7 min and <2 min, respectively). DPP-4 (lymphocyte cell surface protein CD26) is an enzyme present throughout the body cells with highest levels found in the kidney, bone marrow, and intestines.[1]

Gliptins are the class of drugs that work by competitive reversible blockage of the DPP-4 substrate, prolonging the half-life of endogenous GLP-1 and GIP, and increasing their circulating levels. DPP-4 inhibitors at therapeutic doses decrease plasma DPP-4 activity by 70–90% over a sustained period of 24 hours, resulting in (1.5- to 4-fold) increase of GLP-1 levels.[2] DPP-4 inhibitors increase GLP-1 levels, which results in (1) making pancreas to release more insulin in a glucose-dependent fashion in the postprandial phase, thereby decreasing the postprandial glycemic excursions, and (2) slowing of gastric emptying resulting in decreased appetite. The increase in GLP-1 with DPP-4 inhibition is modest and is not as potent as achieved by injection of GLP-1 injection.[2]

There are 11 DPP-4 inhibitors, but only sitagliptin, saxagliptin, linagliptin, and alogliptin are available in the United States. Vildagliptin is available in many other countries, but not in the United States.

Dipeptidyl peptidase-4 inhibitors owing to their structural heterogeneity have a varied pharmacological profile with differences in bioavailability, half-life and mechanism of metabolism, presence of active metabolites, and routes of excretion.[1]

Gliptins have a greater selectivity of 30- to 40,000-fold affinity for DPP-4 enzyme, compared to DPP isozymes such as DPP-8 and DPP-9.[1] DPP-8 and DPP-9 play an important role in immune function by causing T-cell activation and nonselective blockage of DPP-4 inhibitors can potentially cause adverse effects (immune dysfunction, decreased healing, and skin reactions).[2]

Gliptins are well absorbed with oral bioavailability of 75–87%, (except linagliptin which has 30% bioavailability), and absorption is not influenced by food intake.[2]

Linagliptin, alogliptin, and sitagliptin have longer half-lives of 120–184 hours, 12.4–24 hours, and 8–14 hours, respectively. In addition to the longer half-life, these agents cause prolonged DPP-4 enzyme inhibition and are administered as once-a-day medication.[2]

Vildagliptin and saxagliptin half-lives are shorter; 2–3 hours and 2.2–3.8 hours, respectively.[2] As a result of shorter half-life, vildagliptin is administered twice a day. Though saxagliptin has a shorter duration of action, it is also administered as once-a-day regimen, as a major metabolite of saxagliptin is also an active DPP-4 inhibitor which retains about 50% of the DPP-4 inhibition activity.[2]

About 75% of the sitagliptin and 63% of alogliptin are excreted unchanged in the urine.[3]

Vildagliptin is eliminated primarily through hydrolysis in multiple tissues and only one-fourth of the drug is excreted unchanged in the kidneys.[4,5] Saxagliptin unlike other gliptins, is mainly metabolized by cytochrome P450 (CYP)3A4/5 and can potentially cause drug interactions as discussed below.[2] Linagliptin has a unique pharmacokinetic and pharmacodynamic profile and is 99% bound to plasma proteins, mainly to the DPP-4 enzyme (because of nonpolar surface area and its high binding affinity). In virtue of the protein binding property, 80% of the linagliptin is cleared via the enterohepatic system;[2] consequently, it does not require dose adjustment in patients with kidney disease and liver impairment (**Table 5.1**).[1]

TABLE 5.1: List of commonly used gliptins.

Drugs	Brand name	Approval	30-day cost average of highest mg dose in dollars[5]	Dosage forms	Combinations available
Sitagliptin	Januvia	FDA, 2006	457.20	50, 100 mg tablets	Janumet (+metformin) Juvisync (+simvastatin)
Vildagliptin	Galvus	EU, 2007	N/A	50, 100 mg tablets	–
Saxagliptin	Onglyza	FDA, 2009	462.17	2.5, 5 mg tablets	Kombiglyze (+metformin)
Linagliptin	Tradjenta	FDA, 2011	357.20	5 mg tablets	Jentadueto (+metformin)
Alogliptin	Nesina	FDA, 2013	374.20	25 mg tablets	Kazano (+metformin) Oseni (+pioglitazone)
Anagliptin	Suiny	Japan, 2012	N/A	200 mg tablets 400 mg tablets	–
Teneligliptin	Tenelia	Japan, 2012	N/A	20 mg tablets 40 mg tablets	–

(EU: European Union; FDA: Food and Drug Administration)

EFFICACY DATA

The efficacy of gliptins has been studied in numerous randomized placebo-controlled studies and is described below.

Monotherapy

Gliptins when used as monotherapy have modest effects on A1c reduction of up to 0.75% (0.4–1.2%) and postmeal glucose reduction of 25 mg/dL (20–60 mg/dL) and fasting glucose decrease of 18 mg/dL (10–35 mg/dL).

Sitagliptin as Monotherapy

In a 18-week randomized controlled trial (RCT) of 521 patients with diabetes and baseline A1c of 8.1%, placebo-subtracted A1c reduction was 0.60% in the sitagliptin 100 mg group compared to 0.48% in the sitagliptin 200 mg group. Glycemic improvements were more prominent in the subgroup of patients with higher A1c of >9% (A1c reduction of 1.2%). Also, other measures of β-cell function [fasting proinsulin: insulin ratio, homeostasis model assessment (HOMA)] are markedly improved. Gastrointestinal side effects and hypoglycemia incidence were similar between the two groups.[6]

In a 24-week RCT, monotherapy with sitagliptin 100 mg resulted in a placebo-corrected reduction in A1c of 0.79%, with a more pronounced reduction in A1c of 1.52%, in patients with baseline A1c of >9%. While there was no increase in the risk of hypoglycemia with sitagliptin, there was an increase in the risk of gastrointestinal side effects (16% in the sitagliptin group compared to 11% in the placebo group).[7]

Saxagliptin as Monotherapy

Saxagliptin 2.5 mg, 5 mg, and 10 mg were evaluated in a 24-week RCT involving 401 patients with uncontrolled type 2 diabetes mellitus (T2DM) and demonstrated mean A1c reductions of 0.43%, 0.46%, and 0.54%, respectively.[8]

Linagliptin as Monotherapy

In a 24-week RCT, linagliptin monotherapy decreased placebo-corrected A1c of 0.69% with a more prominent improvement in A1c of 1.01% in patients with baseline A1c ≥9.0%. Up to 47.1% of the patients in the linagliptin group had glycated hemoglobin (HbA1c) reduction of ≥0.5% compared to the 19% in the placebo arm.[9]

Vildagliptin as Monotherapy

In a 24-week RCT of 632 newly diagnosed T2DM patients with uncontrolled diabetes (average baseline A1c 8.4%), vildagliptin use showed a modest reduction of A1c of 0.8–0.9%.[10]

Alogliptin as Monotherapy

Alogliptin use (12.5 mg and 25 mg doses) in patients with uncontrolled diabetes resulted in an improvement of A1c of 0.56–0.59%.[11]

COMBINATION TREATMENT WITH GLIPTINS

Sitagliptin has been shown to work in synergy with metformin, sulfonylurea (SU), and thiazolidinedione with an additional reduction in A1c.

Sitagliptin + Metformin

In a RCT with a more extended follow-up period of 104 weeks, the addition of sitagliptin to metformin produced an additional 1.1–1.7% reduction in A1c (better A1c reduction with a higher dose of sitagliptin and metformin).[12]

Sitagliptin + Sulfonylurea

In a 24-week RCT, adding sitagliptin to glimepiride treatment was associated with a 0.74% placebo-corrected reduction in A1c and an increased risk for hypoglycemia compared to placebo (12.2% vs. 1.8%).[13]

Sitagliptin + Thiazolidinediones

The addition of sitagliptin to pioglitazone contributed to an additional A1c reduction of 0.7% compared to the pioglitazone monotherapy. Twice the number of patients in the dual therapy arm achieved the target A1c < 7% compared to the monotherapy arm.[14]

Saxagliptin + Metformin

Saxagliptin addition to metformin resulted in an A1c reduction of 0.78%; 46.5% of the patients reached the goal A1c <7%, whereas metformin monotherapy resulted in A1c reduction of 0.37% and only 30.5% of patients achieved desired A1c of 7%.[15]

Saxagliptin + Thiazolidinediones

The combination of saxagliptin 2.5 and 5 mg with a thiazolidinedione (TZD) showed a decrease in A1c of 0.66% and 0.94%, respectively compared to 0.30% A1c reduction in TZD monotherapy. There was no significant difference between the rates of hypoglycemia in the two different groups.[16]

Saxagliptin + Glyburide

A higher proportion of patients on dual therapy of saxagliptin and glyburide achieved HbA1c <7% (22.4–22.8%) compared to the glyburide group (9.1%).[17]

Saxagliptin + Insulin

In an efficacy and safety clinical study of patients with uncontrolled diabetes, saxagliptin as an add-on treatment to insulin alone or combined with metformin resulted in a greater reduction in A1c.[18]

Linagliptin + Metformin

In a 24-week study, dual therapy with linagliptin with metformin achieved a very impressive reduction in placebo-corrected A1c of –1.7%.[19] In a 2-year, parallel group, and noninferiority study of T2DM patients on metformin, comparing the addition of linagliptin 5 mg daily versus glimepiride 1–4 mg daily, linagliptin was noninferior in glycemic reduction (–0.16%) compared to the addition of glimepiride (–0.36%). Notably, hypoglycemia incidence was five times higher in the glimepiride (36%) compared to the linagliptin group (7%).[20]

Saxagliptin + Dapagliflozin + Metformin

In a study evaluating efficacy of combination therapy with saxagliptin + dapagliflozin + metformin *versus* saxagliptin + metformin *versus* dapagliflozin + metformin, A1c reductions were 1.47%, 0.88%, and 1.20%, respectively; proportion of patients who attained glycemic target of <A1c were 41%, 18%, and 22%, respectively.[21]

Linagliptin + Metformin + Sulfonylurea

The addition of linagliptin to patients on combination treatment with metformin and SU in patients with poorly controlled T2DM (HbA1c 7–10%) resulted in a placebo-corrected HbA1c improvement of 0.62%. Higher rates of symptomatic hypoglycemia (16.7%) were noted with the addition of linagliptin group compared to the placebo (4.8%) (**Table 5.2**).[22-34]

ROLE OF GLIPTINS IN THE MANAGEMENT OF TYPE 2 DIABETES MELLITUS

Current antidiabetic medications such as SU, thiazolidinedione, and insulin cause undesirable weight gain of up to 2 kg for every 1% decrease in the A1c. Reasons for the weight gain are multifactorial, including decrease in metabolic rate, decrease in glycosuria, hypoglycemia episodes resulting in defensive snacking and treatment of hypoglycemia episodes, and an increase in adipose tissue and fluid retention.

Gliptins have a low risk of hypoglycemia and do not cause weight gain, thus offering a favorable side effect profile and can be used as monotherapy or as a combination with other diabetes medications.

TABLE 5.2: Representative studies of gliptins in combination with other agents.

Combination studied	Duration of the study	Intervention	Baseline A1c	Change in HbA1c	Proportion of patients with HbA1c <7%	Comments
Sitagliptin + Metformin[12]	RCT 104 weeks	Sitagliptin 100 mg daily	7.5–11%	–1.2%	32%	• Addition of sitagliptin to metformin did not worsen the gastrointestinal side effects • Low rate of hypoglycemia during the study period
		Metformin 1,000 mg twice a day		–1.3%	45%	
		Metformin 500 mg twice a day		–1.1%	28%	
		Metformin 500 mg bid + Sitagliptin 50 mg bid		–1.4%	45%	
		Metformin 1,000 mg bid + Sitagliptin 50 mg bid		–1.7%	60%	
Sitagliptin + SU[13]	RCT 24 weeks	Glimepiride	8.34%	+0.27%		Higher rates of mild hypoglycemia are noted in patients on a combination of sitagliptin, metformin, and glimepiride
		Glimepiride + Metformin		+0.30%		
		Glimepiride + Sitagliptin 10 mg		–0.27%		
		Glimepiride + Metformin + Sitagliptin 100 mg		–0.59%		
Sitagliptin + thiazolidinediones[14]	RCT 24 weeks	Sitagliptin 100 mg + Pioglitazone 30–45 mg daily	8.1%	–0.15%	45.4%	No increase in hypoglycemia
		Pioglitazone 30–45 mg daily		–0.85%	23%	

Continued

Continued

Combination studied	Duration of the study	Intervention	Baseline A1c	Change in HbA1c	Proportion of patients with HbA1c <7%	Comments
Saxagliptin + thiazolidinediones[16]	RCT 24 weeks	Pioglitazone 30 or 45 mg or rosiglitazone 4 or 8 mg	7–10.5%	–0.30%	25.6%	No significant difference in the rate of hypoglycemia and adverse events
		Pioglitazone 30 or 45 mg or rosiglitazone 4 or 8 mg or saxagliptin 2.5 mg		–0.66%	42.2%	
		Pioglitazone 30 or 45 mg or rosiglitazone 4 or 8 mg + Saxagliptin 5 mg		–0.94%	41.8%	
Saxagliptin + SU[17]	RCT 24 weeks	Glyburide 15 mg/day		+0.08%	9.1%	No significant difference in the rate of hypoglycemia and adverse events
		Glyburide 7.5 mg/day + Saxagliptin 2.5 mg		–0.64%	22.4%	
		Glyburide 7.5 mg/day + Saxagliptin 5 mg		–0.54%	22.8%	
Saxagliptin + Insulin[18]	RCT 24 weeks	Insulin therapy 30–150 U/day ± Metformin		–0.41%		No significant difference in the rate of hypoglycemia
		Insulin therapy 30–150 U/day ± Metformin + Saxagliptin 5 mg daily		–0.80%		

Continued

Continued

Combination studied	Duration of the study	Intervention	Baseline A1c	Change in HbA1c	Proportion of patients with HbA1c <7%	Comments
Linagliptin + Metformin[19]	RCT 24 weeks	Metformin 500 mg bid	8.7%	–0.6%		No significant difference in the rate of hypoglycemia and adverse events
		Metformin 1,000 mg bid		–0.8%		
		Metformin 500 mg bid + Linagliptin 2.5 mg bid		–1.2%		
		Metformin 1,000 mg bid + Linagliptin 2.5 mg bid		–1.7%		
		Linagliptin 5 mg daily		–0.5%		
Saxagliptin + Dapagliflozin + Metformin[21]	RCT 24 weeks	Metformin + Saxagliptin	8.9%	–0.9%	18%	• No significant difference in the rate of hypoglycemia
		Dapagliflozin + Metformin + Saxagliptin		–1.5%	41%	• More UTIs in the dapagliflozin group
Sitagliptin + Insulin[23]	RCT 24 weeks	Insulin ± Metformin	8.7%	0%	13%	Incidence of hypoglycemia was in the sitagliptin group (16%) vs. placebo (8%)
		Insulin + Sitagliptin 100 mg ± Metformin		–0.6%	5%	

Continued

Continued

Combination studied	Duration of the study	Intervention	Baseline A1c	Change in HbA1c	Proportion of patients with HbA1c <7%	Comments
Sitagliptin + SGLT-2[24]	24 weeks RCT followed by 24-week extension	Sitagliptin 100 mg daily	8%	0%	5%	• Genital infection rate in dapagliflozin was high at 9.8% vs. placebo 0.4%
		Dapagliflozin 10 mg/day + Sitagliptin 100 mg daily	7.9%	0.5%	13%	• Dapagliflozin caused more weight loss vs. placebo (–2.1 and –0.3 kg, respectively)
Linagliptin + Thiazolidinediones[25]	RCT 24 weeks	Pioglitazone 30 mg		–0.56%	30.5%	No significant difference in the rate of hypoglycemia and adverse events
		Pioglitazone 30 mg + Linagliptin 5 mg		–1.06%	42.9%	
Linagliptin + Empagliflozin[26]	RCT 52 weeks	Empagliflozin 25 mg	A1c 7.9–8%	–0.95%	41.5%	No significant difference in the rate of hypoglycemia and adverse events
		Empagliflozin 10 mg		–0.83%	38.8%	
		Linagliptin 5 mg		–0.67%	32.3%	
		Empagliflozin 25 mg + Linagliptin 5 mg		–1.08%	62.3%	
		Empagliflozin 10 mg + Linagliptin 5 mg		–1.24%	55.4%	

Continued

Continued

Combination studied	Duration of the study	Intervention	Baseline A1c	Change in HbA1c	Proportion of patients with HbA1c <7%	Comments
Vildagliptin + Metformin[27]	RCT 24 weeks	Vildagliptin 50 mg bid	8.6–8.7%	−1.1%	40%	No significant difference in the rate of hypoglycemia and adverse events
		Metformin 1,000 mg bid		−1.4%	43.5%	
		Metformin 1,000 mg bid + Vildagliptin 50 mg bid		−1.8%	65.4%	
		Metformin 500 mg bid + Vildagliptin 50 mg bid		−1.6%	55.4%	
Vildagliptin + SU[28]	RCT 24 weeks	Glimepiride 4 mg daily	A1c 8.5–8.6%	+0.07%	12%	Vildagliptin 100 mg has a higher hypoglycemia rate (3.6%) than vildagliptin 50 mg (1.2%) or placebo (0.6%)
		Glimepiride 4 mg daily + Vildagliptin 50 mg		−0.58%	21.2%	
		Glimepiride 4 mg daily + Vildagliptin 100 mg		−0.63%	24.8%	
Vildagliptin + Thiazolidinediones[29]	RCT 24 weeks	Pioglitazone 30 mg	A1c 8.6–8.7%	−1.4%	42.9%	Adverse event rates were comparable across treatment arms except pioglitazone monotherapy is associated with a 9.3% risk of peripheral edema
		Vildagliptin 100 mg		−1.1%	42.5%	
		Pioglitazone 30 mg + Vildagliptin 100 mg		−1.9%	65%	
		Pioglitazone 15 mg + Vildagliptin 50 mg		−1.7%	53.6%	

Continued

Continued

Combination studied	Duration of the study	Intervention	Baseline A1c	Change in HbA1c	Proportion of patients with HbA1c <7%	Comments
Vildagliptin + Insulin[30]	RCT 24 weeks	Insulin >30 units	8.4%	–0.2%	NA	Vildagliptin group was associated with lower risk of hypoglycemia
		Insulin >30 units + Vildagliptin 100 mg		–0.5%		
Alogliptin + Pioglitazone[31]	RCT 26 weeks	Pioglitazone 30 or 45 mg	8–8.1%	–0.19%	34%	No significant difference in the rate of hypoglycemia but more cardiac events were noted in the combination group
		Pioglitazone 30 or 45 mg + Alogliptin 12.5 mg		–0.66%	44.2%	
		Pioglitazone 30 or 45 mg + Alogliptin 25 mg		–0.80%	49.2%	
Alogliptin + Metformin[32]	RCT 26 weeks	Metformin	7.9–8%	–0.1%		No significant difference in the rate of adverse events
		Metformin + Alogliptin 12.5 mg		–0.6%		
		Metformin MTD + Alogliptin 25 mg		–0.6%		
Alogliptin+ Glyburide[33]	RCT 26 weeks	Glyburide	8.1%	+0.01%	18.2%	• No significant difference in the rate of hypoglycemia • Higher rate of side effects was noted in the combination group compared to glyburide group
		Glyburide + Alogliptin 12.5 mg		–0.38%	29.6%	
		Glyburide + Alogliptin 25 mg		–0.52%	34.8%	

Continued

Continued

Combination studied	Duration of the study	Intervention	Baseline A1c	Change in HbA1c	Proportion of patients with HbA1c <7%	Comments
Sitagliptin + Metformin + Glimepiride[13]	RCT 24 weeks	Metformin + Glimepiride	8.34%	0.30%	NA	• Sitagliptin has a higher rate of hypoglycemia compared to the control group (12% vs. 2%, respectively) • A mild increase in the weight gain was noted with triple combination therapy compared to placebo (+0.8 kg vs. –0.4 kg)
		Metformin + Glimepiride + Sitagliptin 100 mg		–0.59%		
Alogliptin + Pioglitazone + Metformin[34]	RCT 52 weeks	Metformin + Pioglitazone	8.3%	–0.29%	21.3%	No significant difference in the rate of hypoglycemia and adverse events
		Metformin + Pioglitazone + Alogliptin 25 mg daily		–0.70%	33.2%	

(RCT: randomized controlled trial; SGLT-2: sodium-glucose cotransporter-2; SU: sulfonylurea)

Gliptins have positive effects on β-cell function and are considered a good treatment option early in the course of diabetes, as they have been shown in some studies to preserve β-cell function.

Dipeptidyl peptidase-4 inhibitors are most useful in patients requiring a modest decrease in A1c with a low risk of hypoglycemia.

The selection of the DPP-4 inhibitor is based upon the patient's clinical features, side effects profile, comorbid conditions, insurance cost, and coverage.

Gliptins in Diabetes Management: Guidelines

As per the American Association of Clinical Endocrinologists (AACE) guidelines, DPP-4 can be used as monotherapy in patients with A1c <7.5% or as an add-on agent to other antihyperglycemic agents with A1c >7.5%.

As per the 2019 American Diabetes Association (ADA) guidelines, metformin is the recommended first-line therapy.[35] In patients with atherosclerotic cardiovascular disease or heart failure or chronic kidney disease (CKD), gliptins can be used as an add-on third-line agent to the combination of metformin + sodium-glucose cotransporter-2 (SGLT-2) inhibitors (saxagliptin is not to be used in heart failure). In patients with no preexisting atherosclerotic cardiovascular disease, gliptins can be considered as an add-on second-line agent to metformin and as a third-line agent to metformin + SGLT-2 inhibitor.

Choice of the Agent

In a systemic review evaluating efficacy and safety of gliptins, saxagliptin, sitagliptin, alogliptin, linagliptin, and vildagliptin used either as monotherapy or as dual therapy (in combination with metformin or SU) showed no significant difference in terms of average reduction in HbA1c, the proportion of patients achieving HbA1c <7%, body weight change from baseline, and hypoglycemia rates.[36] Other significant findings from this study are—(1) No significant difference was found in the dual therapy combination treatment of pioglitazone plus gliptins (alogliptin, linagliptin, sitagliptin, and vildagliptin), (2) No difference in the efficacy between the combination therapy with insulin + sitagliptin and insulin + vildagliptin, and (3) No difference between the triple combination group of SU and metformin and gliptins (vildagliptin, sitagliptin, and linagliptin).

Adverse Events

Dipeptidyl peptidase-4 inhibitors were introduced in 2006, and we have 13 years of data about these agents to make generalizations about their side effects.

The risk of hypoglycemia is minimal when used alone or used with metformin. The effects of GLP-1 on insulin secretion are glucose dependent with predominant activity seen only when blood glucose levels are elevated. Hypoglycemia can occur when taking with SU or insulin.

In a systematic review of 67 RCTs, there was an increase in the risk of asthenia [relative risk (RR) 1.53; 95% confidence interval (CI) 1.08–2.16] with vildagliptin and cardiac events (RR 1.37; 95% CI 1–1.89) and vascular disorders (RR 1.74; 95% CI 1.05–2.86) with linagliptin.[37]

Infections

Early studies raised concerns regarding an increase in the risk of infections in patients taking sitagliptin. The findings from a recent meta-analysis are reassuring. Vildagliptin, saxagliptin, linagliptin, or alogliptin use did not increase the incidence of upper respiratory infection or urinary tract infection. Marginally increased risk of nasopharyngitis is noted with sitagliptin (RR 1.3; 95% CI 1.03–1.77).[38]

Cutaneous Reactions

Postmarketing surveillance reported rare cases of severe hypersensitivity skin reactions, including anaphylaxis and angioedema. Vildagliptin was associated with an increased incidence of angioedema in patients receiving angiotensin-converting enzyme (ACE) inhibitors compared with the control group (odds ratio 4.57; 95% CI 1.57–13.28) and it is not clear if this complication is specific to vildagliptin or DPP-4 class effect. However, in various pooled studies, long-term RCTs, and postmarketing safety studies, the incidence of angioedema was not higher with the use of sitagliptin, alogliptin, and saxagliptin compared to placebo.[38]

Pancreatic Adverse Effects[39]

Several case reports were published about DPP-4 inhibitors-associated pancreatitis, but these case reports do not prove gliptins as the cause of acute pancreatitis. In randomized phase 3 clinical trials, a weak signal is noted between gliptin use and pancreatitis, but given the short duration of clinical trials, no clinically significant difference in the incidence of pancreatitis was noted. In the pooled analysis of studies evaluating the cardiovascular safety of gliptins, a large number of patients were monitored over a longer period of time and this allowed for studying the impact of gliptins role in rare adverse events like pancreatitis. In a meta-analysis of three large randomized cardiovascular safety trials, use of gliptins resulted in a 79% increase in RR of acute pancreatitis, but the absolute risk was low at 0.13% (one to two extra cases of acute pancreatitis per 1,000 patients of gliptin use for 2 years).[40] Risk of pancreatic cancer was similar to other diabetes medicines.[37]

Drug–drug Interactions

Gliptins, except saxagliptin and linagliptin, have no significant P450-related metabolism, hence have a low risk of drug-to-drug interactions.

Saxagliptin, unlike other gliptins, is primarily metabolized by the CYP3A4 (cytochrome P450 isoenzyme) and the major metabolite of saxagliptin is also an active DPP-4 inhibitor with about 50% of potency. Therefore, when saxagliptin is administered with strong CYP3A4/5 inhibitors (ketoconazole, clarithromycin, atazanavir, indinavir, itraconazole, nefazodone, ritonavir, nelfinavir, telithromycin, and saquinavir), it can increase the levels of saxagliptin and its active metabolites. Hence, saxagliptin dose should be reduced to 2.5 mg daily when used concomitantly with these medicines.[41] CYP3A4 or P-glycoprotein (P-gp) inducers like rifampin can decrease levels of linagliptin to subtherapeutic concentrations. Therefore, in patients requiring use of such drugs, linagliptin should not be used, and an alternative agent needs to be prescribed.

When gliptins are used along with SU and insulin, dose reduction of SU and insulin might be required to prevent hypoglycemia episodes; this is a pharmacodynamics interaction rather than a pharmacokinetic interaction.

Other than the exceptions detailed above, no significant drug-drug interactions were reported with coadministration of gliptins with commonly prescribed antihyperglycemic medicines, antihypertensive agents, and lipid-lowering medications.

CARDIOVASCULAR SAFETY AND DIPEPTIDYL PEPTIDASE-4 INHIBITORS

In 2008, the Food and Drug Administration (FDA) issued guidance of all new therapies of T2DM that should have a comprehensive evaluation of the cardiovascular safety profile. The following long-term clinical trials were performed to evaluate gliptins safety.

Saxagliptin Assessment of Vascular Outcomes Recorded in Patients with Diabetes Mellitus—Thrombolysis in Myocardial Infarction[42]

In a study of 16,492 patients with T2DM associated with cardiovascular disease, use of saxagliptin was not associated with adverse cardiac outcomes over 2.1 years, except for the slightly higher rate of heart failure hospitalizations in the saxagliptin group (3.5%) compared with placebo (2.8%).

Examination of Cardiovascular Outcomes with Alogliptin versus Standard of Care[43]

In this study of 5,380 patients with T2DM with a recent cardiac event, there was no significant difference in the cardiovascular outcomes between alogliptin and the placebo group.

Vildagliptin in Ventricular Dysfunction Diabetes Study[44]

In this small study of 254 patients with T2DM with heart disease, use of vildagliptin was not associated with any difference in the rate of hospitalization and degree of left ventricular (LV) function, but increase in the end-diastolic volume in the vildagliptin group was noted and the cause and significance of this finding is unknown.

Trial Evaluating Cardiovascular Outcomes with Sitagliptin Study[45]

Safety of sitagliptin was evaluated in 14,671 patients with diabetes and preexisting cardiac disease; at three years, sitagliptin use did not result in an increase in the risk of cardiac events, hypoglycemia rates, and risk of pancreatitis.

Cardiovascular Outcome Study of Linagliptin versus Glimepiride in Patients with Type 2 Diabetes Trial[46]

In this long-term clinical trial (median follow 6.3 years) of patients with diabetes and high cardiovascular disease risk, cardiac outcomes were similar between linagliptin and glimepiride.

A systemic review and meta-analysis of 38 RCTs and 12 observational studies concluded that gliptins are associated with a higher risk of heart failure hospitalizations in patients with preexisting cardiac disease or with several risk factors for vascular disease.[47]

As per the FDA guidance, alogliptin and saxagliptin use in patients with preexisting heart disease or renal disease might increase the risk of heart failure and these agents should be discontinued if patients develop heart failure. The FDA also extended the warning about the risk of heart failure to sitagliptin and linagliptin use.[48]

DIPEPTIDYL PEPTIDASE-4 INHIBITORS IN RENAL AND HEPATIC FUNCTION

Dose modifications that are recommended with kidney and renal disease are summarized in **Table 5.3.**[49,50]

GLIPTINS IN ELDERLY PATIENTS

Elderly patients with diabetes due to associated comorbidities have a higher rate of polypharmacy with a resultant risk of drug-drug interactions. Gliptins are desirable drugs in elderly patients because of their favorable drug interaction profile and low risk of hypoglycemia.

In the TECOS (Trial Evaluating Cardiovascular Outcomes with Sitagliptin) study, sitagliptin use was evaluated in 2,004 patients older than 75 years; sitagliptin use was associated with similar glycemic reductions between older and younger groups, with no increase in the risk of cardiac events, pancreatitis, and hypoglycemia. Patients in this study had a median follow-up of 2.9 years, were attending outpatient clinics every six months, baseline entry A1c was 7.2 (6.5–8%), and patients with estimated glomerular filtration rate (eGFR) <30 mL/min/1.73 m^2 were excluded from this study. Hence, these study findings are not applicable to frail patients with higher A1c and severe CKD and do not inform regarding the long-term safety.[51]

A systemic review on the use of gliptins in elderly concluded that the A1c reduction in elderly patients is similar to younger patients with low risk of hypoglycemia.[52]

In a post-hoc pooled analyses of vildagliptin 100 mg daily monotherapy comparing patients >65 years versus <65 years or as an add-on treatment to metformin in patients >75 years versus <75 years, there was no significant difference in the A1c reductions.[53]

CONCLUSION

In summary, DPP-4 inhibitors offer several advantages such as ease of use (one pill a day), low incidence of hypoglycemia, and are weight neutral drugs. Gliptins cause a modest decrease in A1c of 0.5–1% and have a more significant reduction in A1c, when baseline A1c is higher. Limitations do persist; they only offer a modest lowering of A1c and may not be effective enough in patients with very high A1c to meet the therapeutic goal. Also, the current price of the medicine is in the range of 350–400 dollars/month, and a significant proportion of the patients may not be able to afford them. Caution should be used in using these drugs with preexisting heart failure. Long-term large-scale prospective studies and careful postmarketing surveillance are required to establish the long-term safety of gliptins definitively.

TABLE 5.3: Dose modifications recommended for kidney and renal disease.[4,49,50,]

Drugs	Normal kidney function	Mild CKD and creatinine clearance (50–80)	Moderate CKD and creatinine clearance (30–50)	Severe CKD <30	ESRD	Dose change in hepatic dysfunction
Sitagliptin	100 mg daily	100 mg daily	50 mg daily	25 mg daily	25 mg daily	No dosage adjustment is required for mild-to-moderate hepatic impairment; not studied in severe impairment
Saxagliptin	5 mg daily	5 mg daily	2.5 mg daily	2.5 mg daily (use with caution)	2.5 mg Dose post dialysis (use with caution)	No dose adjustment
Vildagliptin	50 mg bid	50 mg bid	50 mg daily	50 mg daily	50 mg daily (use with caution)	Not recommended for use
Linagliptin	5 mg daily	No dose adjustment	No dose adjustment	No dose adjustment	No dose adjustment	No dose adjustment
Alogliptin	25 mg daily	No dose adjustment	12.5 mg daily	6.25 mg daily	6.25 mg daily	No dosage adjustment is required for mild-to-moderate hepatic impairment; not studied in severe impairment

(CKD: chronic kidney disease; ESRD: end-stage renal disease)

REFERENCES

1. Capuano A, Sportiello L, Maiorino MI, Rossi F, Giugliano D, Esposito K. Dipeptidyl peptidase-4 inhibitors in type 2 diabetes therapy—focus on alogliptin. Drug Des Devel Ther. 2013;7:989-1001.
2. Baetta R, Corsini A. Pharmacology of dipeptidyl peptidase-4 inhibitors: similarities and differences. Drugs. 2011;71:1441-67.
3. Golightly LK, Drayna CC, McDermott MT. Comparative Clinical Pharmacokinetics of Dipeptidyl Peptidase-4 Inhibitors. Clin Pharmacokinet. 2012;51:501-14.
4. Russo E, Penno G, Prato SD. Managing diabetic patients with moderate or severe renal impairment using DPP-4 inhibitors: focus on vildagliptin. Diabetes Metab Syndr Obes. 2013;6:161-70.
5. Munir KM, Lamos EM. Diabetes type 2 management: what are the differences between DPP-4 inhibitors and how do you choose? Exp Opin Pharmacother. 2017;18:839-41.
6. Raz I, Hanefeld M, Xu L, Caria C, Williams-Herman D, Khatami H, et al. Efficacy and safety of the dipeptidyl peptidase-4 inhibitor sitagliptin as monotherapy in patients with type 2 diabetes mellitus. Diabetologia. 2006;49:2564-71.
7. Aschner P, Kipnes MS, Lunceford JK, Sanchez M, Mickel C, Williams-Herman DE, et al. Effect of the dipeptidyl peptidase-4 inhibitor sitagliptin as monotherapy on glycemic control in patients with type 2 diabetes. Diabetes Care. 2006;29:2632-7.
8. Rosenstock J, Aguilar-Salinas C, Klein E, Nepal S, List J, Chen R, et al. Effect of Saxagliptin Monotherapy in Treatment-Naïve Patients With Type 2 Diabetes. Curr Med Res Opin. 2009;25:2401-11.
9. Del Prato S, Barnett AH, Huisman H, Neubacher D, Woerle HJ, Dugi KA. Effect of linagliptin monotherapy on glycaemic control and markers of beta-cell function in patients with inadequately controlled type 2 diabetes: a randomized controlled trial. Diabetes Obes Metab. 2011;13:258-67.
10. Dejager S, Razac S, Foley JE, Schweizer A. Vildagliptin in drug-naïve patients with type 2 diabetes: a 24-week, double-blind, randomized, placebo-controlled, multiple-dose study. Horm Metab Res. 2007;39:218-23.
11. DeFronzo RA, Fleck PR, Wilson CA, Mekki Q, Alogliptin Study 010 Group. Efficacy and safety of the dipeptidyl peptidase-4 inhibitor alogliptin in patients with type 2 diabetes and inadequate glycemic control: a randomized, double-blind, placebo-controlled study. Diabetes Care. 2008;31:2315-7.
12. Williams-Herman D, Johnson J, Teng R, Golm G, Kaufman KD, Goldstein BJ, et al. Efficacy and safety of sitagliptin and metformin as initial combination therapy and as monotherapy over 2 years in patients with type 2 diabetes. Diabetes Obes Metab. 2010;12:442-51.
13. Hermansen K, Kipnes M, Luo E, Fanurik D, Khatami H, Stein P, et al. Efficacy and safety of the dipeptidyl peptidase-4 inhibitor, sitagliptin, in patients with type 2 diabetes mellitus inadequately controlled on glimepiride alone or on glimepiride and metformin. Diabetes Obes Metab. 2007;9:733-45.
14. Rosenstock J, Brazg R, Andryuk PJ, Lu K, Stein P, Sitagliptin Study 019 Group. Efficacy and safety of the dipeptidyl peptidase-4 inhibitor sitagliptin added to ongoing pioglitazone therapy in patients with type 2 diabetes: A 24-week, multicenter, randomized, double-blind, placebo-controlled, parallel-group study. Clin Ther. 2006;28:1556-68.
15. Yang W, Pan CY, Tou C, Zhao J, Gause-Nilsson I. Efficacy and safety of saxagliptin added to metformin in Asian people with type 2 diabetes mellitus: a randomized controlled trial. Diabetes Res Clin Pract. 2011;94:217-24.
16. Hollander P, Li J, Allen E, Chen R, CV181-013 Investigators. Saxagliptin added to a thiazolidinedione improves glycemic control in patients with type 2 diabetes and inadequate control on thiazolidinedione alone. J Clin Endocrinol Metab. 2009;94:4810-9.

17. Chacra AR, Tan GH, Apanovitch A, Ravichandran S, List J, Chen R. Saxagliptin added to a submaximal dose of sulphonylurea improves glycaemic control compared with uptitration of sulphonylurea in patients with type 2 diabetes: a randomized controlled trial. Int J Clin Pract. 2009;63:1395-406.
18. Barnett AH, Charbonnel B, Donovan M, Fleming D, Chen R. Effect of saxagliptin as add-on therapy in patients with poorly controlled type 2 diabetes on insulin alone or insulin combined with metformin. Curr Med Res Opin. 2012;28:513-23.
19. Haak T, Meinicke T, Jones R, Weber S, von Eynatten M, Woerle HJ. Initial combination of linagliptin and metformin improves glycaemic control in type 2 diabetes: a randomized, double-blind, placebo-controlled study. Diabetes Obes Metab. 2012;14:565-74.
20. Gallwitz B, Rosenstock J, Rauch T, Bhattacharya S, Patel S, von Eynatten M, et al. 2-year efficacy and safety of linagliptin compared with glimepiride in patients with type 2 diabetes inadequately controlled on metformin: a randomised, double-blind, non-inferiority trial. Lancet. 2012;380:475-83.
21. Rosenstock J, Hansen L, Zee P, Li Y, Cook W, Hirshberg B, et al. Dual add-on therapy in type 2 diabetes poorly controlled with metformin monotherapy: a randomized double-blind trial of saxagliptin plus dapagliflozin addition vs single addition of saxagliptin or dapagliflozin to metformin. Diabetes Care. 2015;38:376-83.
22. Owens DR, Swallow R, Dugi KA, Woerle HJ. Efficacy and safety of linagliptin in persons with type 2 diabetes inadequately controlled by a combination of metformin and sulphonylurea: a 24-week randomized study. Diabet Med. 2011;28:1352-61.
23. Vilsbøll T, Rosenstock J, Yki-Järvinen H, Cefalu WT, Chen Y, Luo E, et al. Efficacy and safety of sitagliptin when added to insulin therapy in patients with type 2 diabetes. Diabetes Obes Metab. 2010;12:167-77.
24. Jabbour SA, Hardy E, Sugg J, Parikh S, Study 10 Group. Dapagliflozin Is Effective as Add-on Therapy to Sitagliptin With or Without Metformin: A 24-Week, Multicenter, Randomized, Double-Blind, Placebo-Controlled Study. Diabetes Care. 2014;37:740-50.
25. Gomis R, Espadero RM, Jones R, Woerle HJ, Dugi KA. Efficacy and safety of initial combination therapy with linagliptin and pioglitazone in patients with inadequately controlled type 2 diabetes: a randomized, double-blind, placebo-controlled study. Diabetes Obes Metab. 2011;13:653-61.
26. Lewin A, DeFronzo RA, Patel S, Liu D, Kaste R, Woerle HJ, et al. Initial combination of empagliflozin and linagliptin in subjects with type 2 diabetes. Diabetes Care. 2015;38:394-402.
27. Bosi E, Dotta F, Jia Y, Goodman M. Vildagliptin plus metformin combination therapy provides superior glycaemic control to individual monotherapy in treatment-naive patients with type 2 diabetes mellitus. Diabetes Obes Metab. 2009;11:506-15.
28. Garber AJ, Foley JE, Banerji MA, Ebeling P, Gudbjornsdottir S, Camisasca RP, et al. Effects of vildagliptin on glucose control in patients with type 2 diabetes inadequately controlled with a sulphonylurea. Diabetes Obes Metab. 2008;10:1047-56.
29. Rosenstock J, Kim SW, Baron MA, Camisasca RP, Couturier A, Dejager S. Efficacy and tolerability of initial combination therapy with vildagliptin and pioglitazone compared with component monotherapy in patients with type 2 diabetes. Diabetes Obes Metab. 2007;9:175-85.
30. Fonseca V, Schweizer A, Albrecht D, Baron MA, Chang I, Dejager S. Addition of Vildagliptin to Insulin Improves Glycaemic Control in Type 2 Diabetes. Diabetologia. 2007;50:1148-55.
31. Pratley RE, Reusch JEB, Fleck PR, Wilson CA, Mekki Q, Alogliptin Study 009 Group. Efficacy and safety of the dipeptidyl peptidase-4 inhibitor alogliptin added to pioglitazone in patients with type-2 diabetes: a randomized, double-blind, placebo-controlled study. Curr Med Res Opin. 2009;25:2361-71.

32. Nauck MA, Ellis GC, Fleck PR, Wilson CA, Mekki Q, Alogliptin Study 008 Group. Efficacy and safety of adding the dipeptidyl peptidase-4 inhibitor alogliptin to metformin therapy in patients with type-2 diabetes inadequately controlled with metformin monotherapy: a multicentre, randomized, double-blind, placebo-controlled study. Int J Clin Pract. 2009;63:46-55.
33. Pratley RE, Kipnes MS, Fleck PR, Wilson C, Mekki Q, Alogliptin Study 007 Group. Efficacy and safety of the dipeptidyl peptidase-4 inhibitor alogliptin in patients with type-2 diabetes inadequately controlled by glyburide monotherapy. Diabetes Obes Metab. 2009;11:167-76.
34. Bosi E, Ellis GC, Wilson CA, Fleck PR. Alogliptin as a third oral antidiabetic drug in patients with type 2 diabetes and inadequate glycemic control on metformin and pioglitazone: a 52-week, randomized, double-blind, active-controlled, parallel-group study. Diabetes Obes Metab. 2011;13:1088-96.
35. American Diabetes Association. Pharmacologic Approaches to Glycemic Treatment: Standards of Medical Care in Diabetes—2019. Diabetes Care. 2019;42:S90-102.
36. Craddy P, Palin HJ, Johnson KI. Comparative effectiveness of dipeptidyl peptidase-4 inhibitors in type 2 diabetes: a systematic review and mixed treatment comparison. Diabetes Ther. 2014;5:1-41.
37. Goοßen K, Gräber S. Longer term safety of dipeptidyl peptidase-4 inhibitors in patients with type 2 diabetes mellitus: systematic review and meta-analysis. Diabetes Obes Metab. 2012;14:1061-72.
38. Karagiannis T, Boura P, Tsapas A. Safety of dipeptidyl peptidase 4 inhibitors: a perspective review. Ther Adv Drug Saf. 2014;5:138-46.
39. DeVries JH, Rosenstock J. DPP-4 Inhibitor-Related Pancreatitis: Rare but Real! Diabetes Care. 2017;40:161-3.
40. Tká I, Raz I. Combined analysis of three large interventional trials with gliptins indicates increased incidence of acute pancreatitis in patients with type 2 diabetes. Diabetes Care. 2017;40:284-6.
41. Food and Drug Administration (FDA). (2017). Onglyza® (saxagliptin). [online] Available from https://www.azpicentral.com/onglyza/onglyza.pdf. [Last accessed February, 2020].
42. Scirica BM, Bha DL, Braunwald E, Steg PG, Davidson J, Hirshberg B, et al. Saxagliptin and cardiovascular outcomes in patients with type 2 diabetes mellitus. N Engl J Med. 2013;369:1317-26.
43. White WB, Bakris GL, Bergenstal RM, Cannon CP, Cushman WC, Fleck P, et al. Examination of cardiovascular outcomes with alogliptin versus standard of care in patients with type 2 diabetes mellitus and acute coronary syndrome (EXAMINE): A cardiovascular safety study of the dipeptidyl peptidase 4 inhibitor alogliptin in patients with type 2 diabetes mellitus with acute coronary syndrome. Am Heart J. 2011;162:620-6.e1.
44. McMurray JJV, Ponikowski P, Bolli GB, Lukashevich V, Kozlovski P, Kothny W, et al. Effects of Vildagliptin on Ventricular Function in Patients With Type 2 Diabetes Mellitus and Heart Failure: A Randomized Placebo-Controlled Trial. JACC Heart Fail. 2018;6:8-17.
45. Green JB, Bethel MA, Armstrong PW, Buse JB, Engel SS, Garg J, et al. Effect of sitagliptin on cardiovascular outcomes in type 2 diabetes. N Engl J Med. 2015;373:232-42.
46. Rosenstock J, Kahn SE, Johansen OE, Zinman B, Espeland MA, Woerle HJ, et al. Effect of Linagliptin vs Glimepiride on Major Adverse Cardiovascular Outcomes in Patients With Type 2 Diabetes: The CAROLINA Randomized Clinical Trial. JAMA. 2019;322:1155-66.
47. Li L, Li S, Deng K, Liu J, Vandvik PO, Zhao P, et al. Dipeptidyl peptidase-4 inhibitors and risk of heart failure in type 2 diabetes: systematic review and meta-analysis of randomised and observational studies. BMJ. 2016;352:i610.
48. Food and Drug Administration (FDA). (2019). FDA Drug Safety Communication: FDA adds warnings about heart failure risk to labels of type 2 diabetes medicines containing saxagliptin and alogliptin. [online] Available from

https://www.fda.gov/drugs/drug-safety-and-availability/fda-drug-safety-communication-fda-adds-warnings-about-heart-failure-risk-labels-type-2-diabetes. [Last accessed February, 2020].
49. Scheen AJ. A review of gliptins in 2011. Exp Opin Pharmacother. 2012;13:81-99.
50. Scheen AJ. Pharmacokinetics of dipeptidyl peptidase-4 inhibitors. Diabetes Obes Metab. 2010;12:648-58.
51. Bethel MA, Engel SS, Green JB, Huang Z, Josse RG, Kaufman KD, et al. Assessing the Safety of Sitagliptin in Older Participants in the Trial Evaluating Cardiovascular Outcomes With Sitagliptin (TECOS). Diabetes Care. 2017;40: 494-501.
52. Schwartz SL. Treatment of elderly patients with type 2 diabetes mellitus: a systematic review of the benefits and risks of dipeptidyl peptidase-4 inhibitors. Am J Geriatr Pharmacother. 2010;8:405-18.
53. Pratley RE, Rosenstock J, Pi-Sunyer FX, Banerji MA, Schweizer A, Couturier A, et al. Management of type 2 diabetes in treatment-naive elderly patients: benefits and risks of vildagliptin monotherapy. Diabetes Care. 2007;30:3017-22.

6
CHAPTER

Glucagon-like Peptide-1 Receptor Agonists for Type 2 Diabetes Mellitus

Arti Bhan, Rebecca Marie Simon

INTRODUCTION

An estimated 382 million people worldwide are affected by diabetes with 30 million affected in the United States and approximately 72 million in India, with type 2 diabetes mellitus (T2DM) comprising over 95% of all diagnosed cases.[1,2] Guidelines for management of T2DM recommend a patient-centered approach to treatment, with individualized glycemic targets, minimizing the risk of hypoglycemia and preventing complications.[3]

Lifestyle modifications and metformin are the first-line treatment modalities for T2DM. Second-line treatment entails the addition of another oral agent, a glucagon-like peptide-1 receptor agonist (GLP-1 RA) or insulin therapy.[4] In patients intolerant to metformin, GLP-1 RAs can be used as first line agents. The choice of GLP-1 RA depends on several factors, including efficacy of the agent to lower glycated hemoglobin (HbA1c), patient preference, side effect profile, risk of hypoglycemia, and effects on weight and cost. In a systematic review of patient preferences for noninsulin diabetes medications, weight loss and glycemic control were the two most important factors driving patient preferences.[5] GLP-1 RA can be used as components of dual or triple therapy regimens and is attractive, as they confer not only consistent glycemic control and weight loss, but also protection against hypoglycemia. Furthermore, GLP-1 RA can also be used as an alternative to basal insulin for certain patients, since they provide at least similar efficacy without weight gain and, in most cases, a lower risk of hypoglycemia.[6]

BACKGROUND

Incretin hormones are released in a biphasic manner from the gastrointestinal tract in response to ingestion of nutrients and they stimulate insulin secretion by the pancreatic β-cells and suppress glucagon secretion.[7] There are two naturally occurring incretins that play an important role in the maintenance of glycemic control—(1) glucose-dependent insulinotropic polypeptide (GIP) and (2) glucagon-like peptide-1 (GLP-1). Both types of incretins have short half-lives due to rapid degradation by dipeptidyl peptidase-4 (DPP-4) enzyme. In patients with T2DM, the effect of incretins is attenuated or even absent.[8] The administration of pharmacological doses of GLP-1 restores insulin secretion by the β cell and this was the basis for the development of GLP-1 receptor agonists.[9]

Glucagon-like peptide-1 has the following multiple physiological effects that play a complementary role in glucose homeostasis:[10]

- Stimulation of insulin secretion by the β cell in a glucose-dependent manner
- Suppression of glucagon release from the α cell in the presence of high glucose
- Reduce hepatic glucose output
- Delay gastric emptying
- Promote satiety via central neural mechanisms.

Also, in animal models, GLP-1 has been shown to promote β-cell growth and inhibit apoptosis.[11] GLP-1 RAs have molecular structures and incretin effect similar to native GLP-1, but are resistant to degradation by DPP-4.

Currently, there are six different GLP-1 RA available for clinical use and differ from each other by molecular structure and size, duration of action, pharmacokinetics, ability to penetrate different tissue compartments, dosing frequency, HbA1c lowering ability, and side effect profiles (**Table 6.1**).

In the upcoming section, we will discuss salient details of each GLP-1 RA.

EXENATIDE

This is a synthetic version of exendin-4, a peptide found in the saliva of the Gila monster.[12] It has about 50% molecular homology with the mammalian GLP-1. It is the first Food and Drug Administration (FDA) approved GLP-1 RA and has a half-life of 2.4 hours after subcutaneous administration, thus requiring twice daily dosing. The duration of exenatide in the circulation is approximately 10 hours. Exenatide is available in either 5 or 10 μg doses given subcutaneously within 1 hour of the morning and evening meals.

Exenatide has greater effects on postprandial glucose excursion than fasting glucose levels, probably because of its short half-life. Exenatide also promotes weight loss with a mean decrease of approximately 1.5–3.7 kg in clinical trials (**Fig. 6.1**).[13,14]

TABLE 6.1: Dosing, titration, and administration recommendations for glucagon-like peptide-1 (GLP-1) receptor agonists.

Drug names	Frequency given	Relation to meals	Initial dose and titration	Recommended final dose
Exenatide	Twice daily	Within 60 min before main meal	5 µg twice daily before meals for 1 month	10 µg BID
Liraglutide	Once daily	Inject any time	0.6 µg once daily for 1 week	1.2–1.8 µg once daily
Lixisenatide	Once daily	Within 60 min before any meal	10 µg once daily for 2 weeks	20 µg once daily
Exenatide LAR	Once weekly	Inject any time	No titration	2 µg once weekly
Dulaglutide	Once weekly	Inject any time	No titration	0.75–1.5 mg once weekly
Semaglutide	Once weekly	Inject any time	0.25 mg once weekly for 4 weeks	0.5–1.0 mg once weekly

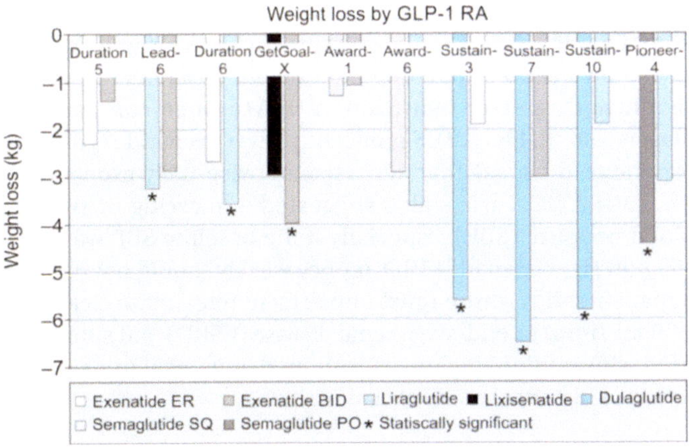

Above data is based on 10 head-to-head clinical trials comparing different GLP-1 RAs. Statistically significant differences between groups are denoted by.

(AWARD: Assessment of Weekly Administration of Dulaglutide in Diabetes; DURATION: Diabetes Therapy Utilization: Researching Changes in A1c, Weight and Other Factors through Intervention with Exenatide Once Weekly; GLP-1: glucagon-like peptide-1; LEAD-6: Liraglutide Effect and Action in Diabetes 6; SUSTAIN: Semaglutide Unabated Sustainability in Treatment of Type 2 Diabetes; PIONEER-4: Peptide Innovation for Early Diabetes Treatment)

FIG. 6.1: Weight loss with various GLP-1 receptor agonists (RAs) in head-to-head clinical trials.

The AMIGO (AC2993 Diabetes Management for Improving Glucose Outcomes) trials were three 30-week randomized, triple-blind, and placebo-controlled trials that examined the effect of exenatide treatment on glycemic control in patients with T2DM. In the AMIGO trials, patients were randomized to placebo, exenatide 5 µg or 10 µg, while continuing metformin and/or sulfonylurea. At the end of the studies, HbA1c reductions of 0.8–1.5% from baseline were achieved.[15-17]

Exenatide is generally well tolerated with mild-to-moderate gastrointestinal effects being the most common adverse effect. A gradual dose escalation helps ameliorate some of these effects, especially nausea and vomiting. Exenatide twice daily has also been compared to glargine or biphasic insulin aspart in two open label trials in patients with inadequately controlled diabetes on metformin. Results showed similar reductions in HbA1c with improved weight loss and less nocturnal hypoglycemia.[18,19] In combination with basal insulin therapy, exenatide demonstrated a significant improvement in reduction in HbA1c as compared with placebo (–0.96% vs. –0.23%) in patients with T2DM inadequately controlled on glargine.

Exenatide QW is the same molecule found in exenatide BID, except that it is formulated in microspheres to provide extended release. The half-life of exenatide QW is greater than a week. A series of phase III trials, collectively referred to as the DURATION (Diabetes Therapy Utilization: Researching Changes in A1c, Weight and Other Factors through Intervention with Exenatide Once Weekly) trials, showed HbA1c reductions of 1.2–1.9% with similar effects on weight loss as twice-daily exenatide (**Fig. 6.1**).[20-23] The sustained-release formulation has also shown success in combination with basal insulin with a significantly greater reduction in HbA1c when compared to placebo alone (**Fig. 6.2**). Significantly fewer exenatide QW users experienced nausea than did users of twice-daily exenatide.[23] The DURATION trials also suggested a lowering of systolic blood pressure (SBP), especially if the baseline SBP was over 130 mm Hg.[22] Exenatide BID or once weekly should not be used in patients with severe renal impairment (creatinine clearance < 30 mL/min) or end-stage renal disease (ESRD) and should be used with caution in patients with moderate renal impairment or with a history of renal transplantation.

LIRAGLUTIDE

This is a synthetic GLP-1 and has 97% homology with human GLP-1. The addition of a fatty acid side chain enables once a day dosing by prolonging its duration of action to over 24 hours.[24] Liraglutide has a better effect on fasting glucose compared to postprandial glucose. It is dosed as 0.6 mg once daily for the first week and is increased to 1.2 mg once daily thereafter.

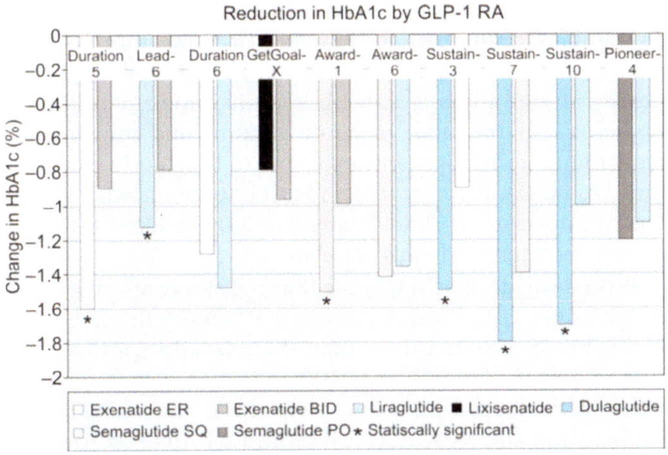

Above data is based on 10 head-to-head clinical trials comparing different GLP-1 RAs. Statistically significant differences between groups are denoted by.

(AWARD: Assessment of Weekly Administration of Dulaglutide in Diabetes; DURATION: Diabetes Therapy Utilization: Researching Changes in A1c, Weight and Other Factors through Intervention with Exenatide Once Weekly; GLP-1: glucagon-like peptide-1; HbA1c: glycated hemoglobin; LEAD-6: Liraglutide Effect and Action in Diabetes 6; SUSTAIN: Semaglutide Unabated Sustainability in Treatment of Type 2 Diabetes; PIONEER-4: Peptide Innovation for Early Diabetes Treatment)

FIG. 6.2: Reduction in glycated hemoglobin (HbA1c) by GLP-1 receptor agonists (RAs).

If blood sugars remain uncontrolled, liraglutide can eventually be titrated to 1.8 mg once daily. Liraglutide was studied as monotherapy and in combination with other agents used to treat T2DM in six randomized, controlled phase III trials known as the LEAD (Liraglutide Effect and Action in Diabetes) program. The trial included over 4,000 patients in 40 countries. In these studies, liraglutide led to improvement in glycemic control. As monotherapy, liraglutide lowered HbA1c by 0.84% and by 1.14% with the 1.2 mg and 1.8 mg doses, respectively (**Fig. 6.2**).[25] When added to one or two oral antidiabetic agents, liraglutide reduced HbA1c by 1.1–1.5%.[26-28] Liraglutide has also been shown to have a protective effect on renal function. The LEADER-RENAL study showed that among patients who were receiving usual care, liraglutide resulted in significantly lower rates of renal outcomes than placebo among patients with T2DM who were at high cardiovascular risk. This was mostly due to a lower incidence of macroalbuminuria in the liraglutide group compared to the placebo group. The risk of doubling of serum creatinine level and of ESRD was also lower in the liraglutide group, although it did not achieve statistical significance.[29]

Liraglutide is also formulated in combination with insulin degludec as Xultophy. In one trial, patients uncontrolled on metformin and glargine were randomized to further glargine titration versus degludec-liraglutide and outcomes demonstrated a greater A1c reduction in the degludec-liraglutide group (–1.8% vs. –1.1%) and a greater weight loss.[30] Liraglutide can be used in patients with severe renal impairment [estimated glomerular filtration rate (eGFR)[3] 15 to <30 mL/min/1.73 m^2] without dose adjustment. The pharmacokinetics of liraglutide may be altered in patients with hepatic impairment due to the binding of liraglutide to serum albumin and concomitant hypoalbuminemia. Systemic exposure to liraglutide has been found to be significantly lower (44%) in patients with severe hepatic impairment (Child–Pugh score >9); therefore, this drug is not recommended in this population.[31]

The 3.0-mg dose of liraglutide (Saxenda) was first approved in December 2014 for the treatment of obesity in the United States, being a higher dose than that already approved for second-line treatment of T2DM.[32] The FDA approval for Saxenda was based on results from three phase III clinical trials called the SCALE (Satiety and Clinical Adiposity-Liraglutide Evidence) studies, which were conducted to evaluate the efficacy and safety of the drug.[33,34] The three studies enrolled >5,000 participants who were obese or overweight and with or without weight-related conditions. The study results demonstrated that patients treated with liraglutide experienced statistically significant reduction in weight, compared to placebo after 56 weeks. It is approved by the FDA for adult patients with a body mass index (BMI) greater than 30 kg/m^2 alone or greater than 27 kg/m^2 in the presence of at least one weight-related comorbidity, such as hypertension, diabetes, or dyslipidemia.

DULAGLUTIDE

This is a long-acting GLP-1 RA, formulated for once-weekly subcutaneous administration, with a half-life of 5 days. The molecule comprises two GLP-1 analog chains linked to an immunoglobulin G fragment, forming a large molecule that has slower absorption and a reduced rate of renal clearance and degradation by DPP-4.[35] Therapeutic concentrations are achieved faster with dulaglutide compared to other once-weekly GLP-1 analogs within 1–3 days.

Dulaglutide is dosed at 0.75 mg once weekly and can be administered at any time of the day. After 6–8 weeks, the dose can be increased to 1.5 mg once weekly if glucose values are not controlled. Missed doses should be administered within 3 days of the missed dose. No dose adjustment is needed for patients with mild, moderate, or severe renal impairment. Dulaglutide demonstrated glycemic efficacy in a variety of phase III trials collectively known as the AWARD (Assessment of Weekly Administration of Dulaglutide in Diabetes) studies which included over 5,000 patients.[36,37] Active comparators included exenatide twice daily, insulin glargine, and liraglutide, in conjunction with background treatment with metformin, pioglitazone, and insulin, depending on study design. As monotherapy, dulaglutide at both the 0.75 mg and 1.5 mg dose was shown to be superior to metformin with a significant improvement in weight loss as well (**Figs. 6.1** and **6.2**). Dulaglutide has also been compared to glargine in patients with moderate-to-severe kidney disease in the AWARD-7 trial and shown to produce better glycemic control.[38] In the AWARD-4 trial, dulaglutide at both doses had a statistically significant improvement in HbA1c reduction (–1.42% and –1.48% vs. –1.23%) compared to glargine in patients already treated with prandial lispro with or without metformin.[39] Adverse effects of dulaglutide are comparable to other GLP-1 RAs with nausea, vomiting, and diarrhea being the most commonly reported side effects.

Lixisenatide is a GLP-1 RA, which has a shorter half-life of 3 hours. The initial dose is 10 μg administered once daily prior to any meal which can be increased to 20 μg daily after a couple weeks of use. Lixisenatide has been studied as monotherapy, in combination with oral antidiabetic medications, and in combination with basal insulin and all have been shown a significant reduction in HbA1c.[40-42] Efficacy of lixisenatide in T2DM has been compared with placebo, exenatide, and glulisine. In comparison with placebo, lixisenatide has shown a greater reduction in A1c when added to metformin (–0.9% vs. –0.4% with placebo) (**Fig. 6.2**) In a 24-week noninferiority trial, lixisenatide was found to be noninferior in comparison with exenatide when adding onto metformin in patients with inadequately controlled T2DM (A1c reduction of –0.79% vs. –0.96% with exenatide).[41] Multiple studies have shown improvement in A1c of patients given lixisenatide when inadequately controlled on glargine and metformin. Lixisenatide can also be found in combination with glargine under the brand name Soliqua. No dose adjustment is needed in patients with renal insufficiency.

Semaglutide is a GLP-1 RA with an extended half-life of approximately 1 week and is thus dosed once weekly for subcutaneous administration or once daily in its oral form. The increase in half-life of this drug is due to its affinity to bind with albumin. Subcutaneous semaglutide is dosed initially as 0.25 mg once weekly and increased after 4 weeks to 0.5 mg once weekly. If glucose levels remain above goal at this dose, it can be increased to 1 mg once weekly after another 4 weeks. The SUSTAIN (Semaglutide Unabated Sustainability in Treatment of Type 2 Diabetes) is the clinical trial program which looked the safety and efficacy of semaglutide in combination with placebo and other diabetes medications. The SUSTAIN-1 trial showed semaglutide as monotherapy to have a mean A1c reduction around –1.5% compared to –0.02% in the placebo group and also resulted in significant weight loss between 3.7 kg and 4.5 kg depending on the dose used.[43] In comparison with glargine as an add-on to metformin in the SUSTAIN-4 trial, semaglutide at both 0.5 and 1 mg dosing resulted in significantly greater reductions in HbA1c compared with glargine (–1.2%, –1.6%, and –0.8%, respectively).[44] Mean body weight decreased by 3.5–5.2 kg in the semaglutide arm (**Figs. 6.1** and **6.2**). The SUSTAIN-6 trial was a cardiovascular safety study for the drug and noted increase in rates of retinopathy which has not been clearly explained though suspected to be related to a rapid drop in glucose levels. Therefore, it is recommended to titrate the medication up slowly, especially in patients with known retinopathy.[45]

Semaglutide is the first in the class of GLP-1 RA available for oral administration thereby making it attractive to patients and clinicians and may promote earlier initiation of appropriate therapy. As compared to the injectable preparation, oral semaglutide has a different absorption profile but once absorbed, the pharmacokinetic properties and effects are similar, regardless of the route of administration. Oral semaglutide is dosed once a day and is approved in two dose formulations, 7 mg and 14 mg, with a starter dose of 3 mg prescribed for the first 30 days. The medication is administered 30 minutes prior to the first meal of the day, with no >4 ounces of water. Oral semaglutide was compared with placebo and subcutaneous semaglutide in patients with T2DM. Over a 26-week period, oral semaglutide resulted in HbA1c reduction of 0.7–1.9% compared to placebo and weight reduction in the range of 2.1–6.9 kg.[46] The PIONEER-1 study also showed superiority of monotherapy with oral semaglutide over placebo, with nausea being the main adverse effect.[47] Oral semaglutide has a cardiovascular safety profile similar to that of the subcutaneous form.[48] Gastrointestinal side effects were the main reason for drug discontinuation in the PIONEER-6 study.

INDICATIONS FOR TREATMENT

All GLP-1 RAs are indicated in combination with other glucose-lowering medications including insulin. Liraglutide, dulaglutide, and semaglutide are also indicated as monotherapy, after lifestyle modifications are not sufficient for control and metformin therapy is considered inappropriate, due to side effects or contraindications. All GLP-1 RAs can be used with metformin and/or sulfonylureas. When adding a GLP-1 RA to a regimen containing sulfonylurea, consider lowering the dose of sulfonylurea to reduce the risk of hypoglycemia. DPP-4 inhibitors should not be used with GLP-1 RAs. When adding a GLP-1 RA to basal insulin, it is recommended that the dose of insulin be reduced to reduce the risk of hypoglycemia. However, this does not apply to exenatide QW. The initial dose reduction can be up to 20% for patients with an A1c of less than 8%. Dose reduction is not necessary when A1c is high. Only dulaglutide has data showing safety with prandial insulin but GLP-1 RAs have been used in clinical settings with basal and prandial insulin.[39]

CARDIOVASCULAR SAFETY OF GLUCAGON-LIKE PEPTIDE-1 RECEPTOR AGONISTS

Patients with T2DM are at increased risk for cardiovascular disease (CVD). Compared to people without diabetes, the incidence of myocardial infarctions, strokes, coronary death, peripheral vascular disease, and heart failure are all increased in people with diabetes. In 2017, the total cost of diagnosed diabetes in the United States was $327 billion and CVD is the largest contributor to the direct and indirect costs of diabetes.[49] Since 2008, in the wake of concerns about the CV safety of the thiazolidinedione and rosiglitazone, the USFDA issued guidance that all drugs investigated for diabetes should be evaluated for cardiovascular effects.[50] Phase II and III trials are now required to demonstrate cardiovascular safety, especially in patients with advanced age and renal dysfunction. In addition to improving glucose control, GLP-1 RAs have shown a benefit in CVD outcomes, particularly liraglutide, semaglutide, and dulaglutide (**Table 6.2**).[45,51,52]

In a trial of 9,340 patients with T2DM and coexisting CVD or at least one cardiovascular risk factor, patients were randomized to subcutaneous liraglutide or placebo in addition to other oral diabetes agents and insulin. Rates of death from cardiovascular cause, nonfatal myocardial infarction (MI), and nonfatal stroke were significantly less likely in the liraglutide group (13% vs. 14.9%). These patients also had a lower HbA1c, weight, and SBP.[53] Similarly, semaglutide was compared to placebo in the SUSTAIN-6 trial which included 3,297 patients with established CVD or age >50 years with at least one risk factor for CVD. These patients were followed for 2 years with a significantly lower rate of cardiovascular-related death, nonfatal MI, and nonfatal stroke in the semaglutide group (6.6% vs. 8.9%). In addition to improvement in HbA1c, there was a reduction in SBP and weight. Finally, dulaglutide is the third GLP-1 RA found to improve CVD outcomes in a trial of 9,901 patients with established CVD or risk factors. After a 5.4-year follow-up, death from cardiovascular causes, nonfatal MI, and nonfatal stroke was significantly lower in the dulaglutide group compared to placebo.[52] There was also a greater reduction in HbA1c, weight, and SBP in this group when comparing to placebo. Lixisenatide and extended-release exenatide were also evaluated and both had no significant difference in cardiovascular outcomes in comparison with placebo.[54] GLP-1 RAs have been shown to decrease SBP and to a lesser extent, diastolic blood pressure (DBP). This class of drugs has also been shown to have a salutary effect on lipid profiles

TABLE 6.2: Summary of cardiovascular outcome trials for each GLP-1 receptor agonist drug. All drugs showed noninferiority compared to usual care. Liraglutide, semaglutide, and dulaglutide had a significant reduction in major adverse cardiovascular event (MACE) as well as significant renal benefit. Liraglutide also showed a significant reduction in all-cause mortality.

	ELIXA Lixisenatide n = 6,068	LEADER Liraglutide n = 9,340	SUSTAIN-6 Semaglutide n = 3,297	EXCEL Exenatide n = 14,752	REWIND Dulaglutide n = 9,901
Primary endpoint	CV death, nonfatal MI, and nonfatal stroke	CV death, nonfatal MI, or nonfatal stroke	CV death, nonfatal MI, or nonfatal stroke	CV death, nonfatal MI, or nonfatal stroke	CV death, nonfatal MI, or nonfatal stroke
Median follow-up (years)	2.1	3.8	2.1	3.2	5.4
Intervention	Lixisenatide 20 µg vs. usual care	Liraglutide 1.8 mg vs. usual care	Semaglutide 0.5 or 1 mg versus usual care	Exenatide ER 2 mg vs. usual care	Dulaglutide 1.5 mg vs. usual care
Noninferiority compared to usual care	Yes	Yes	Yes	Yes	Yes
Significant reduction in MACE (primary endpoint)	No	Yes	Yes	No	Yes
All-cause mortality reduction	No	Yes	No	No	No
Significant renal benefit	No	Yes	Yes	No	Yes

(ELIXA: Evaluation of Lixisenatide in Acute Coronary Syndrome; EXCEL: Evaluation of XIENCE versus Coronary Artery Bypass Surgery for Effectiveness of Left Main Revascularization; GLP-1: glucagon-like peptide-1; LEADER: Liraglutide Effect and Action in Diabetes: Evaluation of Cardiovascular Outcome Results; MI: myocardial infarction; SUSTAIN-6: Semaglutide Unabated Sustainability in Treatment of Type 2 Diabetes-6) with studies showing a significant reduction in low-density lipoprotein (LDL) cholesterol.[55]

SAFETY CONSIDERATIONS AND SIDE EFFECTS

Almost all the drugs belonging to group GLP-1 RAs are usually tolerated to a good extent. Frequent unfavorable effects of the drugs include mild-to-moderate nausea and vomiting. The side effects are temporary and the patients are able to tolerate these adverse effects in a period of time. The occurrence of nausea varies with intake of each drug of this class—13% with dulaglutide (0.75 mg), about 20% with liraglutide, exenatide QW, dulaglutide (1.5 mg) and semaglutide, and as high as 26% with lixisenatide and 36% with exenatide once every day. Patients discontinuing the intake of drug because of the nausea and vomiting and adverse effects seem very less, approximately 1% with prolonged-release exenatide to a maximum of 5% with semaglutide and once-daily exenatide. This group of drugs should ideally be avoided in patients with gastroparesis as it extents the time of gastric emptying.

Even though no cases of medullary thyroid carcinoma have been reported in clinical trials of GLP-1 RA, these medications are contraindicated in patients with a personal or family history of medullary thyroid carcinoma and patients with multiple endocrine neoplasia type 2.

Occasionally, the adverse effects nausea and vomiting, may lead to severe dehydration and renal impairment.[56] In such cases, maintaining hydration is recommended. In diabetic retinopathy patients, administering insulin in combination with semaglutide has been shown to enhance the susceptibility of retinopathy complications.[45] Hence, administering insulin along with semaglutide in diabetic retinopathy cases requires utmost caution.

There have been reports of acute pancreatitis associated with GLP-1 RAs, but insufficient data to determine a causal relationship and the overall incidence is quite low, cited at 16 patients out of over 14,000 patients in one meta-analysis.[57] These medications should be avoided in patients with a prior history of pancreatitis and should be used with caution in those who are at high risk for developing pancreatitis.

SUMMARY

Agents in the GLP-1 RA class are effective treatment options for patients with T2DM, offering many advantages over other agents, including weight loss, potential β-cell protection, and low risk of hypoglycemia, in addition to improving glycemic control. This class of drugs also has positive benefits on cardiovascular parameters including a reduction in blood pressure, lipids, and body weight. These medications are available in various dosing modalities ranging from twice-daily injections to weekly injections and now an oral formulation as well. This translates to better patient satisfaction and thereby adherence to treatment. These agents can be combined with a variety of antidiabetes medications and can safely be used as monotherapy or add-on treatment for a durable response.

REFERENCES

1. Centers for Disease Control and Prevention (CDC). (2017). National Diabetes Statistics Report, 2017: Estimates of Diabetes and its Burden in the United States. [online] Available from https://www.cdc.gov/diabetes/pdfs/data/statistics/national-diabetes-statistics-report.pdf. [Last accessed February, 2020].
2. Anjana RM, Pradeepa R, Deepa M, Datta M, Sudha V, Unnikrishnan R, et al. The Indian Council of Medical Research-India Diabetes (ICMR-INDIAB) study: methodological details. J Diabetes Sci Technol. 2011;5(4):906-14.
3. Inzucchi SE, Bergenstal RM, Buse JB, Diamant M, Ferrannini E, Nauck M, et al. Management of hyperglycemia in type 2 diabetes, 2015: a patient-centered approach: update to a position statement of the American Diabetes Association and the European Association for the Study of Diabetes. Diabetes Care. 2015;38(1):140-9.
4. American Diabetes Association. 9. Pharmacologic Approaches to Glycemic Treatment: Standards of Medical Care in Diabetes-2019. Diabetes Care. 2019;42(Suppl 1):S90-102.
5. Purnell TS, Joy S, Little E, Bridges JF, Maruthur N. Patient preferences for noninsulin diabetes medications: a systematic review. Diabetes Care. 2014;37(7):2055-62.
6. Amori RE, Lau J, Pittas AG. Efficacy and safety of incretin therapy in type 2 diabetes: systematic review and meta-analysis. JAMA. 2007;298(2):194-206.
7. Baggio LL, Drucker DJ. Biology of incretins: GLP-1 and GIP. Gastroenterology. 2007;132(6):2131-57.
8. Holst JJ, Knop FK, Vilsboll T, Krarup T, Madsbad S. Loss of incretin effect is a specific, important, and early characteristic of type 2 diabetes. Diabetes Care. 2011;34 Suppl 2:S251-7.
9. Nauck MA, Bartels E, Orskov C, Ebert R, Creutzfeldt W. Additive insulinotropic effects of exogenous synthetic human gastric inhibitory polypeptide and glucagon-like peptide-1-(7-36) amide infused at near-physiological insulinotropic hormone and glucose concentrations. J Clin Endocrinol Metab. 1993;76(4):912-7.
10. Zander M, Madsbad S, Madsen JL, Holst JJ. Effect of 6-week course of glucagon-like peptide 1 on glycaemic control, insulin sensitivity, and beta-cell function in type 2 diabetes: a parallel-group study. Lancet. 2002;359(9309):824-30.
11. Aaboe K, Krarup T, Madsbad S, Holst JJ. GLP-1: physiological effects and potential therapeutic applications. Diabetes Obes Metab. 2008;10(11):994-1003.
12. Eng J, Kleinman WA, Singh L, Singh G, Raufman JP. Isolation and characterization of exendin-4, an exendin-3 analogue, from Heloderma suspectum venom. Further evidence for an exendin receptor on dispersed acini from guinea pig pancreas. J Biol Chem. 1992;267(11):7402-5.
13. Buse JB, Klonoff DC, Nielsen LL, Guan X, Bowlus CL, Holcombe JH, et al. Metabolic effects of two years of exenatide treatment on diabetes, obesity, and hepatic biomarkers in patients with type 2 diabetes: an interim analysis of data from the open-label, uncontrolled extension of three double-blind, placebo-controlled trials. Clin Ther. 2007;29(1):139-53.

14. Riddle MC, Henry RR, Poon TH, Zhang B, Mac SM, Holcombe JH, et al. Exenatide elicits sustained glycaemic control and progressive reduction of body weight in patients with type 2 diabetes inadequately controlled by sulphonylureas with or without metformin. Diabetes Metab Res Rev. 2006;22(6):483-91.
15. DeFronzo RA, Ratner RE, Han J, Kim DD, Fineman MS, Baron AD. Effects of exenatide (exendin-4) on glycemic control and weight over 30 weeks in metformin-treated patients with type 2 diabetes. Diabetes Care. 2005;28(5):1092-100.
16. Buse JB, Henry RR, Han J, Kim DD, Fineman MS, Baron AD, et al. Effects of exenatide (exendin-4) on glycemic control over 30 weeks in sulfonylurea-treated patients with type 2 diabetes. Diabetes Care. 2004;27(11):2628-35.
17. Kendall DM, Riddle MC, Rosenstock J, Zhuang D, Kim DD, Fineman MS, et al. Effects of exenatide (exendin-4) on glycemic control over 30 weeks in patients with type 2 diabetes treated with metformin and a sulfonylurea. Diabetes Care. 2005;28(5):1083-91.
18. Heine RJ, Van Gaal LF, Johns D, Mihm MJ, Widel MH, Brodows RG, et al. Exenatide versus insulin glargine in patients with suboptimally controlled type 2 diabetes: a randomized trial. Ann Intern Med. 2005;143(8):559-69.
19. Nauck MA, Duran S, Kim D, Johns D, Northrup J, Festa A, et al. A comparison of twice-daily exenatide and biphasic insulin aspart in patients with type 2 diabetes who were suboptimally controlled with sulfonylurea and metformin: a non-inferiority study. Diabetologia. 2007;50(2):259-67.
20. Kim D, MacConell L, Zhuang D, Kothare PA, Trautmann M, Fineman M, et al. Effects of once-weekly dosing of a long-acting release formulation of exenatide on glucose control and body weight in subjects with type 2 diabetes. Diabetes Care. 2007;30(6):1487-93.
21. Diamant M, Van Gaal L, Stranks S, Northrup J, Cao D, Taylor K, et al. Once weekly exenatide compared with insulin glargine titrated to target in patients with type 2 diabetes (DURATION-3): an open-label randomised trial. Lancet. 2010;375(9733):2234-43.
22. Diamant M, Van Gaal L, Guerci B, Stranks S, Han J, Malloy J, et al. Exenatide once weekly versus insulin glargine for type 2 diabetes (DURATION-3): 3-year results of an open-label randomised trial. Lancet Diabetes Endocrinol. 2014;2(6):464-73.
23. Bergenstal RM, Wysham C, Macconell L, Malloy J, Walsh B, Yan P, et al. Efficacy and safety of exenatide once weekly versus sitagliptin or pioglitazone as an adjunct to metformin for treatment of type 2 diabetes (DURATION-2): a randomised trial. Lancet. 2010;376(9739):431-9.
24. Elbrond B, Jakobsen G, Larsen S, Agerso H, Jensen LB, Rolan P, et al. Pharmacokinetics, pharmacodynamics, safety, and tolerability of a single-dose of NN2211, a long-acting glucagon-like peptide 1 derivative, in healthy male subjects. Diabetes Care. 2002;25(8):1398-404.
25. Garber A, Henry R, Ratner R, Garcia-Hernandez PA, Rodriguez-Pattzi H, Olvera-Alvarez I, et al. Liraglutide versus glimepiride monotherapy for type 2 diabetes (LEAD-3 Mono): a randomised, 52-week, phase III, double-blind, parallel-treatment trial. Lancet. 2009;373(9662):473-81.
26. Zinman B, Gerich J, Buse JB, Lewin A, Schwartz S, Raskin P, et al. Efficacy and safety of the human glucagon-like peptide-1 analog liraglutide in combination with metformin and thiazolidinedione in patients with type 2 diabetes (LEAD-4 Met+TZD). Diabetes Care. 2009;32(7):1224-30.
27. Russell-Jones D, Vaag A, Schmitz O, Sethi BK, Lalic N, Antic S, et al. Liraglutide vs insulin glargine and placebo in combination with metformin and sulfonylurea therapy in type 2 diabetes mellitus (LEAD-5 met+SU): a randomised controlled trial. Diabetologia. 2009;52(10):2046-55.
28. Buse JB, Rosenstock J, Sesti G, Schmidt WE, Montanya E, Brett JH, et al. Liraglutide once a day versus exenatide twice a day for type 2 diabetes: a

26-week randomised, parallel-group, multinational, open-label trial (LEAD-6). Lancet. 2009;374(9683):39-47.

29. Mann JFE, Ørsted DD, Brown-Frandsen K, Marso SP, Poulter NR, Rasmussen S, et al. Liraglutide and Renal Outcomes in Type 2 Diabetes. N Engl J Med. 2017;377(9):839-48.
30. Lingvay I, Pérez Manghi F, Garcia-Hernández P, Norwood P, Lehmann L, Tarp-Johansen MJ, et al. Effect of Insulin Glargine Up-titration vs Insulin Degludec/Liraglutide on Glycated Hemoglobin Levels in Patients With Uncontrolled Type 2 Diabetes: The DUAL V Randomized Clinical Trial. JAMA. 2016;315(9):898-907.
31. European Medicines Agency. (2018). Victoza: Summary of Product Characteristics. [online] Available from https://www.ema.europa.eu/en/medicines/human/EPAR/victoza. [Last accessed February, 2020].
32. Astrup A, Rossner S, Van Gaal L, Rissanen A, Niskanen L, Al Hakim M, et al. Effects of liraglutide in the treatment of obesity: a randomised, double-blind, placebo-controlled study. Lancet. 2009;374(9701):1606-16.
33. Davies MJ, Bergenstal R, Bode B, Kushner RF, Lewin A, Skjoth TV, et al. Efficacy of Liraglutide for Weight Loss Among Patients With Type 2 Diabetes: The SCALE Diabetes Randomized Clinical Trial. JAMA. 2015;314(7):687-99.
34. Overgaard RV, Petri KC, Jacobsen LV, Jensen CB. Liraglutide 3.0 mg for Weight Management: A Population Pharmacokinetic Analysis. Clin Pharmacokinet. 2016;55(11):1413-22.
35. Barrington P, Chien JY, Showalter HD, Schneck K, Cui S, Tibaldi F, et al. A 5-week study of the pharmacokinetics and pharmacodynamics of LY2189265, a novel, long-acting glucagon-like peptide-1 analogue, in patients with type 2 diabetes. Diabetes Obes Metab. 2011;13(5):426-33.
36. Dungan KM, Povedano ST, Forst T, Gonzalez JG, Atisso C, Sealls W, et al. Once-weekly dulaglutide versus once-daily liraglutide in metformin-treated patients with type 2 diabetes (AWARD-6): a randomised, open-label, phase 3, non-inferiority trial. Lancet. 2014;384(9951):1349-57.
37. Wysham C, Blevins T, Arakaki R, Colon G, Garcia P, Atisso C, et al. Efficacy and safety of dulaglutide added onto pioglitazone and metformin versus exenatide in type 2 diabetes in a randomized controlled trial (AWARD-1). Diabetes Care. 2014;37(8):2159-67.
38. Tuttle KR, Lakshmanan MC, Rayner B, Busch RS, Zimmermann AG, Woodward DB, et al. Dulaglutide versus insulin glargine in patients with type 2 diabetes and moderate-to-severe chronic kidney disease (AWARD-7): a multicentre, open-label, randomised trial. Lancet Diabetes Endocrinol. 2018;6(8):605-17.
39. Blonde L, Jendle J, Gross J, Woo V, Jiang H, Fahrbach JL, et al. Once-weekly dulaglutide versus bedtime insulin glargine, both in combination with prandial insulin lispro, in patients with type 2 diabetes (AWARD-4): a randomised, open-label, phase 3, non-inferiority study. Lancet. 2015;385(9982):2057-66.
40. Ahren B, Leguizamo Dimas A, Miossec P, Saubadu S, Aronson R. Efficacy and safety of lixisenatide once-daily morning or evening injections in type 2 diabetes inadequately controlled on metformin (GetGoal-M). Diabetes Care. 2013;36(9):2543-50.
41. Rosenstock J, Raccah D, Koranyi L, Maffei L, Boka G, Miossec P, et al. Efficacy and safety of lixisenatide once daily versus exenatide twice daily in type 2 diabetes inadequately controlled on metformin: a 24-week, randomized, open-label, active-controlled study (GetGoal-X). Diabetes Care. 2013;36(10):2945-51.
42. Riddle MC, Forst T, Aronson R, Sauque-Reyna L, Souhami E, Silvestre L, et al. Adding once-daily lixisenatide for type 2 diabetes inadequately controlled with newly initiated and continuously titrated basal insulin glargine: a 24-week, randomized, placebo-controlled study (GetGoal-Duo 1). Diabetes Care. 2013;36(9):2497-503.
43. Sorli C, Harashima SI, Tsoukas GM, Unger J, Karsbol JD, Hansen T, et al. Efficacy and safety of once-weekly semaglutide monotherapy versus placebo in patients with type 2 diabetes (SUSTAIN 1): a double-blind, randomised, placebo-controlled, parallel-group, multinational, multicentre phase 3a trial. Lancet Diabetes Endocrinol. 2017;5(4):251-60.

44. Aroda VR, Bain SC, Cariou B, Piletic M, Rose L, Axelsen M, et al. Efficacy and safety of once-weekly semaglutide versus once-daily insulin glargine as add-on to metformin (with or without sulfonylureas) in insulin-naive patients with type 2 diabetes (SUSTAIN 4): a randomised, open-label, parallel-group, multicentre, multinational, phase 3a trial. Lancet Diabetes Endocrinol. 2017;5(5):355-66.
45. Marso SP, Bain SC, Consoli A, Eliaschewitz FG, Jodar E, Leiter LA, et al. Semaglutide and Cardiovascular Outcomes in Patients with Type 2 Diabetes. N Engl J Med. 2016;375(19):1834-44.
46. Davies M, Pieber TR, Hartoft-Nielsen ML, Hansen OKH, Jabbour S, Rosenstock J. Effect of Oral Semaglutide Compared With Placebo and Subcutaneous Semaglutide on Glycemic Control in Patients With Type 2 Diabetes: A Randomized Clinical Trial. JAMA. 2017;318(15):1460-70.
47. Aroda VR, Rosenstock J, Terauchi Y, Altuntas Y, Lalic NM, Morales-Villegas EC, et al. PIONEER 1: Randomized Clinical Trial of the Efficacy and Safety of Oral Semaglutide Monotherapy in Comparison With Placebo in Patients With Type 2 Diabetes. Diabetes Care. 2019;42(9):1724-32.
48. Husain M, Birkenfeld AL, Donsmark M, Dungan K, Eliaschewitz FG, Franco DR, et al. Oral Semaglutide and Cardiovascular Outcomes in Patients with Type 2 Diabetes. N Engl J Med. 2019;381(9):841-51.
49. American Diabetes Association. Economic Costs of Diabetes in the U.S. in 2017. Diabetes Care. 2018;41(5):917-28.
50. U.S. Department of Health and Human Services, Food and Drug Administration. (2008). Guidance for Industry: Diabetes Mellitus—Evaluating Cardiovascular Risk in New Antidiabetic Therapies to Treat Type 2 Diabetes. [online] Available from https://www.fda.gov/media/71297/download. [Last accessed February, 2020].
51. Marso SP, Daniels GH, Brown-Frandsen K, Kristensen P, Mann JF, Nauck MA, et al. Liraglutide and Cardiovascular Outcomes in Type 2 Diabetes. N Engl J Med. 2016;375(4):311-22.
52. Gerstein HC, Colhoun HM, Dagenais GR, Diaz R, Lakshmanan M, Pais P, et al. Dulaglutide and cardiovascular outcomes in type 2 diabetes (REWIND): a double-blind, randomised placebo-controlled trial. Lancet. 2019;394(10193):121-30.
53. Marre M, Shaw J, Brandle M, Bebakar WM, Kamaruddin NA, Strand J, et al. Liraglutide, a once-daily human GLP-1 analogue, added to a sulphonylurea over 26 weeks produces greater improvements in glycaemic and weight control compared with adding rosiglitazone or placebo in subjects with Type 2 diabetes (LEAD-1 SU). Diabet Med. 2009;26(3):268-78.
54. Pfeffer MA, Claggett B, Diaz R, Dickstein K, Gerstein HC, Kober LV, et al. Lixisenatide in Patients with Type 2 Diabetes and Acute Coronary Syndrome. N Engl J Med. 2015;373(23):2247-57.
55. Sun F, Wu S, Wang J, Guo S, Chai S, Yang Z, et al. Effect of glucagon-like peptide-1 receptor agonists on lipid profiles among type 2 diabetes: a systematic review and network meta-analysis. Clin Ther. 2015;37(1):225-41.e8.
56. Filippatos TD, Panagiotopoulou TV, Elisaf MS. Adverse Effects of GLP-1 Receptor Agonists. Rev Diabet Stud. 2014;11(3-4):202-30.
57. Li L, Shen J, Bala MM, Busse JW, Ebrahim S, Vandvik PO, et al. Incretin treatment and risk of pancreatitis in patients with type 2 diabetes mellitus: systematic review and meta-analysis of randomised and non-randomised studies. BMJ. 2014;348:g2366.

7

CHAPTER

Insulin Sensitizers

Ambrish Mithal, Parjeet Kaur

INTRODUCTION

Insulin resistance in muscle, liver, and adipocytes along with β-cell failure are the principal pathophysiologic defects in type 2 diabetes mellitus (T2DM). Two classes of drugs improve insulin action as their key effect: (1) Biguanides; and (2) Thiazolidinediones (TZDs).

Thiazolidinediones were introduced in the late 1990s and troglitazone was the first drug in this class to be marketed. Troglitazone was removed from the market in 2000 due to risk of hepatotoxicity. Currently, rosiglitazone and pioglitazone are available for clinical use in USA, however, rosiglitazone has been removed from the market or its use is restricted in various other countries because of cardiovascular safety concerns.[1] Pioglitazone is currently available for clinical use in several countries, except in France and Germany.

Despite all the safety concerns, TZDs still have a role in management of T2DM, since this is the only class of drugs that predominantly targets insulin resistance. In addition, pioglitazone also has a favorable effect on diabetes prevention and lipid parameters. The mechanism of action, pharmacology, and clinical use of TZDs will be reviewed in this chapter.

MECHANISM OF ACTION

Thiazolidinediones bind to and activate one or more peroxisome proliferator-activated receptors (PPARs). PPARs are nuclear receptors which act as ligand-activated transcription factors. Three isoforms for these receptors have been described: α, β/δ, and γ. PPAR-α is expressed mostly in liver, heart, skeletal muscle, and vascular walls where it plays an important role in fatty acid oxidation. PPAR-γ balances adipogenesis, insulin sensitivity, and lipid metabolism of entire body. Accordingly, it is prevalently seen in adipose tissue, pancreatic β-cells, vascular endothelium, macrophages, and the central nervous system (CNS). TZDs attach to PPAR receptors causing generation of heterodimers with retinoid X receptors (RXRs). In turn, the dimers attach to specific deoxyribonucleic acid (DNA) sequences called as peroxisome proliferator response elements (PPREs), which trigger or hamper the transcription of target genes.

The concentration of PPAR-γ is increased in the skeletal muscle of obese and diabetic patients, where TZDs increase insulin sensitivity by binding to PPAR-γ receptor which results in increase expression of glucose transporter type 4 (GLUT4).[2] Additionally, in human adipocytes, PPAR-γ controls the expression of numerous factors secreted from adipose tissue, such as adiponectin, resistin, leptin, and tumor necrosis factor-α (TNF-α), which also influence insulin sensitivity. Binding of TZDs to PPAR-γ in human adipocytes leads to increase expression of genes involved in promoting lipid storage and decreased expression of genes associated with inflammation such as interleukin-6 (IL-6) and TNF-α, thereby, improving insulin sensitivity.[3] Rosiglitazone is a pure PPAR-γ agonist, while pioglitazone exerts some PPAR-α effects as well, which may explain the different effects that pioglitazone and rosiglitazone have on lipids and cardiovascular ischemic outcomes.

Thiazolidinediones have also been shown to have direct protective effects on β-cells. β-cells express PPAR-γ and PPAR-γ agonist exposure prevents amyloid-induced apoptosis in cultured β-cells.[4] Furthermore, in different animal models of diabetes, TZD treatment resulted in preservation of the pancreatic islets structure and β-cell function.

GLYCEMIC EFFICACY

Thiazolidinediones are potent insulin sensitizers and result in ~0.5–1.4% reduction in glycated hemoglobin (HbA1c) when used as monotherapy.[5] In addition to use as monotherapy, TZDs have been studied in combination with metformin, sulfonylureas, dipeptidyl peptidase-4 (DPP-4) inhibitors, glucagon-like peptide-1 (GLP-1) receptor agonists, sodium-glucose cotransporter-2 (SGLT-2) inhibitors, and insulin. The ADOPT (A Diabetes Outcome Progression Trial) trial investigated the durability of the antihyperglycemic effects of rosiglitazone in drug-naïve patients.[6] Over a period of 4 years, patients who were administered rosiglitazone encountered considerably increased longevity of continuously optimal fasting plasma glucose levels; however, the differences in the glycemic control achievable with rosiglitazone or metformin were small. Glycemic control achieved by TZD was found to be long lasting and could be attained at significantly least risk of hypoglycemia; hence it was recommended as good as other treatment methods. The American Diabetes Association (ADA) recommends use of TZD as a second-line drug in combination with metformin if glycemic target was not achieved with metformin alone.[5]

In addition to increasing insulin sensitivity, TZDs also exert β-cell protective effects which make this the only class of antidiabetic drugs that correct the main defects of insulin resistance and β-cell failure in T2DM. Both pioglitazone and rosiglitazone have been shown to reduce impaired glucose tolerance (IGT) conversion to T2DM.[7,8]

BENEFITS BEYOND GLYCEMIC CONTROL

Effects on the Liver

One of the major etiologies of development of nonalcoholic steatohepatitis (NASH) was found to be insulin resistance. TZDs have insulin-sensitizing property thereby, becoming the recommended drug of choice for treating this disease. The PIVENS (Pioglitazone, Vitamin E, or Placebo for Nonalcoholic Steatohepatitis) trial observed that administering pioglitazone in histologically confirmed NASH patients showed great amounts of lowering in steatosis, inflammation, and hepatocellular ballooning in the absence of diabetes or cirrhosis.[9] On the other hand, trials that used rosiglitazone clinically did not show positive results.

Effects on Restenosis after Percutaneous Transluminal Coronary Angioplasty

Several trials have been performed to investigate the effect of TZDs on restenosis in vessels treated by percutaneous transluminal coronary angioplasty (PTCA). Two meta-analyses performed in patients after coronary stents were placed showed that TZD use considerably decreased the susceptibility of in-stent restenosis, reduced stenosis diameter, delayed loss of lumen, and target vessel revascularization in both diabetic and nondiabetic patients.[10,11] Results with pioglitazone use are more favorable as compared with rosiglitazone. Possible mechanism includes antiproliferative effects of pioglitazone occurring concurrently with its anti-inflammatory action.

SAFETY

Cardiovascular Effects

Effect on Lipids

Effects of pioglitazone and rosiglitazone on serum lipid concentrations are different which may depend upon the specificity of PPAR activation. Effect of pioglitazone on lipid profile has been found favorable in most randomized trials. In a review of six randomized trials, pioglitazone treatment did not change the low-density lipoprotein cholesterol (LDL-C) levels, while rise in LDL-C levels ranging from 8 to 16% were noted in studies of rosiglitazone.[12] Pioglitazone treatment has been shown to decrease triglycerides and produce favorable changes in LDL particle size and concentration in plasma. Both drugs increase high-density lipoprotein cholesterol (HDL-C) levels but increase in HDL levels is reported more with pioglitazone than with rosiglitazone.

Major Cardiovascular Events

Several meta-analyses looking at rosiglitazone use and cardiovascular risk have reported a significant increase in the risk of myocardial infarction (MI) or cardiovascular death or no evidence of effects on MI and other adverse outcomes (morbidity, mortality, and quality of life). The majority of the above studies were not designed to explore cardiovascular outcomes.[1,13,14] Two trials, however, were designed to specifically evaluate cardiovascular outcomes: The RECORD (Rosiglitazone Evaluated for Cardiac Outcomes and Regulation of Glycaemia in Diabetes) study was designed to evaluate the effects of rosiglitazone on cardiovascular events and mortality in 4,447 patients from Europe and Australia.[15] A persistent increased risk of fatal and nonfatal heart failure was noted in rosiglitazone group as opposed to the control group [hazard ratio (HR) 2.10; 95% confidence interval (CI) 1.35–3.27]. The influence of rosiglitazone on MI could not be arrived at exactly due to very few events recorded. With the observation from all the analyses, the Food and Drug Administration (FDA) took off restrictions on rosiglitazone as per the opinion of an expert panel (FDA, 2013). This conclusion was backed by the BARI 2D (The Bypass Angioplasty Revascularization Investigation 2 Diabetes) trial, post hoc analysis, where it was clarified that patients treated with rosiglitazone did not show considerable alteration in MI.[16]

Pioglitazone, on the other hand, may not have the same cardiovascular risk profile as rosiglitazone. A meta-analysis was performed about the use of pioglitazone and cardiovascular safety which presented a considerable 18% lowered susceptibility of composite of cardiovascular events apart from a non-significant tendency for a decreased susceptibility of MI.[17] The PROactive (Prospective Pioglitazone Clinical Trial in Macrovascular Events) trial was specifically designed to evaluate cardiovascular outcomes and presented a very low percentage, 10% decrease in the primary composite endpoint (all-cause mortality, nonfatal MI, acute coronary syndrome, stroke, revascularization of coronary or leg arteries, and amputation above the ankle), and a considerable 16% lowering in the vital prespecified secondary composite endpoint (all-cause mortality, nonfatal MI, and stroke).[18]

Fluid Retention and Heart Failure

Fluid retention can occur with all the TZDs and is more prominent with concomitant insulin therapy. Peripheral edema occurs in 4–6% of patients treated with TZDs.[12] Excess fluid can lead to exacerbations of congestive heart failure (CHF). One of the mechanisms of fluid retention with TZD seems to be PPAR-γ stimulation of sodium reabsorption by sodium channels in the luminal membrane of the collecting tubule cells. TZD induced increased vascular permeability and vasodilatation also contributes to edema.[19]

Rosiglitazone and pioglitazone both increase the CHF events, but do not appear to increase mortality from CHF.[20]

Weight Gain

Several studies have reported weight gain of ~5 kg associated with TZD usage over 3–5 years. TZD-induced weight gain is both dose- and time-dependent.[21] Fluid retention accounts for part of weight gain; however, proliferation of new adipocytes contributes significantly to weight gain.[22] Increase in fat deposition occurs primarily in subcutaneous fat stores, resulting in a decreased visceral-to-subcutaneous fat ratio. In addition, weight gain may be due to TZD induced activation of PPAR-γ in the CNS which has shown to cause increased feeding and expanded adipose tissue mass in animal studies.[23]

Skeletal Fractures

Randomized controlled trials (RCTs) of both pioglitazone and rosiglitazone have shown increased fracture risk particularly in women. However, the fractures did not occur at characteristically osteoporotic sites including spine and hip, but occurred as distal fractures in the upper and lower extremities.[24-27] Pioglitazone decreases the density and content of bone minerals at numerous areas among both genders.

The pathophysiology of skeletal effects of TZDs is still debatable and seems to show both reduced actions of osteoblasts and enhanced actions of osteoclasts. A hypothesis postulates that stimulation of PPAR-γ2 causes deviation of mesenchymal precursor cells away from the osteoblast lineage toward adipocyte lineage, thereby, causing reduction in bone formation rates and high levels of adipogenesis consequently.[28,29] Studies of TZD-induced skeletal effects are also complicated by the fact that diabetes effects bone itself, as patients with diabetes have a higher risk of fracture independent of bone density.

Bladder Cancer

There are several epidemiological studies in humans indicating that pioglitazone increases bladder cancer risk.[30-32] In the French retrospective cohort study of ~1.5 million patients, the risk of bladder cancer increased with high cumulative dose and long duration of exposure (>24 months; HR 1.36; 95% CI 1.04–1.79).[31] In June 2011, administration of pioglitazone was stopped by the French and German Medicines Agencies due to the high susceptibility to bladder cancer. Two subsequent meta-analyses of cohort studies found a similar increased risk of bladder cancer with pioglitazone use.[33,34] A recently published UK cohort study of 145,806 patients found an increased risk of bladder cancer with pioglitazone use (HR 1.63; 95% CI 1.22–2.19). Latest addition to this controversial issue is the meta-analysis which showed that overall relative risk (RR) of bladder cancer with pioglitazone use was as low as 1.13 with 95% CI (0.96–1.33).[35,36] This was associated with decreased heterogeneity in RR studies, thereby proving that using pioglitazone does not have any association increased risk of bladder cancer. The USFDA in 2016 stated that pioglitazone may be linked to an increased risk for bladder cancer. There are no data linking rosiglitazone to bladder cancer.

There is no clarity in the proposed mechanisms of enhanced susceptibility of bladder malignancy in subjects administered with pioglitazone. TZDs are shown to change expansion of tumor in PPAR-γ-independent[37] and PPAR-γ-dependent ways. An alternative mechanism involves alteration of urine composition following treatment, resulting in urinary solids that lead to mucosal irritation and tumors in rats.[38]

Macular Edema

Some studies have shown an association between TZD use and diabetic macular edema and patients at greatest risk seem to be those who are also at risk for peripheral edema.

Hepatotoxicity

Troglitazone was removed from the market due to the reports of severe hepatic toxicity. Trials with rosiglitazone and pioglitazone have shown minor elevations in alanine aminotransferase levels and no patients had values >8–10 times the upper limit of normal.[39,40] However, severe hepatic toxicity has occasionally been reported in patients receiving rosiglitazone or pioglitazone.[41] The FDA currently recommends baseline testing followed by periodic monitoring of liver function based upon clinical judgment in patients receiving pioglitazone or rosiglitazone.

CLINICAL USE

The ADA places TZDs among the second-line agents as an add-on to metformin to achieve glycemic control. However, due to safety concerns, TZDs should be used in selected patients who do not reach glycemic goals with other antidiabetic drugs and where patient preference limits the use of insulin. TZDs use should be avoided under following situations:

- In the presence of significant or proven cardiac disease.
- Symptomatic heart failure or the New York Heart Association class III or IV heart failure.
- Active bladder cancer or history of bladder cancer and discontinue in case when hematuria or any other symptom of bladder cancer develops.
- History of fracture or at high-risk for fracture (e.g., post-menopausal women with low bone mass).
- Active liver disease (liver enzymes >2.5 times above the upper reference limit).
- In patients who are struggling with their weight or need to lose weight.
- In patients with macular edema.

DOSING AND MONITORING

Pioglitazone is usually initiated at a dose of 15 mg daily. Dose can be increased after 2–3 weeks if glycemic control was not achieved to the maximum dose of 45 mg daily. Rosiglitazone is usually initiated at a dose of 4 mg daily and the dose can be increased after 8–12 weeks if the glycemic response is inadequate, to a maximum of 8 mg daily (single daily dose or in divided doses twice daily). TZDs are excreted in the bile either unchanged or as metabolites and eliminated in the feces. No dose adjustment is required in patients with renal impairment; however, TZDs use is avoided in renal impairment due to risk of fluid retention. Dose of TZDs should be gradually escalated. Monitoring for adverse effects should include: Signs and symptoms of heart failure, pedal edema, symptoms that may indicate liver injury (e.g., dark urine, jaundice, right upper abdominal discomfort), and hematuria or any other symptom of bladder cancer.

CONCLUSION

Thiazolidinediones are potent insulin sensitizers that act by binding to nuclear receptor PPAR-γ. TZDs increase insulin sensitivity by acting on adipose, muscle, and liver to increase glucose utilization and decrease glucose production. Anti-hyperglycemic effect of TZD is noninferior to other treatment strategies and is long lasting. In addition, TZDs have been shown to reduce IGT conversion to T2DM. However, use of TZDs is limited by several side effects. Both rosiglitazone and pioglitazone increase the risk of heart failure. However, rosiglitazone use has been associated with a greater risk of adverse cardiovascular events (stroke, heart failure, and all-cause mortality) than pioglitazone. The effect of rosiglitazone on MI remains inconclusive. There is evidence to suggest that TZDs decrease bone density and increase fracture risk, especially in women. The association of bladder cancer with TZD use is controversial; however, there is concern that pioglitazone use increases the risk of bladder cancer. Other adverse effects include weight gain and fluid retention. Despite this, TZDs still have a role in the treatment of T2DM since this is the only class of drugs that primarily targets insulin resistance. Development of newer PPAR agonists with superior benefit-risk balance remains a valuable and promising approach.

REFERENCES

1. Nissen SE, Wolski K. Effect of rosiglitazone on the risk of myocardial infarction and death from cardiovascular causes. N Engl J Med. 2007;356:2457-71.
2. Park KS, Ciaraldi TP, Abrams-Carter L, Mudaliar S, Nikoulina SE, Henry RR. PPAR-gamma gene expression is elevated in skeletal muscle of obese and type II diabetic subjects. Diabetes. 1997;46:1230-4.
3. Sharma AM, Staels B. Review: Peroxisome proliferator-activated receptor gamma and adipose tissue—understanding obesity-related changes in regulation of lipid and glucose metabolism. J Clin Endocrinol Metab. 2007;92:386-95.
4. Dubois M, Pattou F, Kerr-Conte J, Gmyr V, Vandewalle B, Desreumaux P, et al. Expression of peroxisome proliferator-activated receptor gamma (PPARgamma) in normal human pancreatic islet cells. Diabetologia. 2000;43:1165-9.
5. American Diabetes Association. Standards of Medical Care in Diabetes-2017. Diabetes Care. 2017;40:S1-138.
6. Kahn SE, Haffner SM, Heise MA, Herman WH, Holman RR, Jones NP, et al. Glycemic durability of rosiglitazone, metformin, or glyburide monotherapy. N Engl J Med. 2006;355:2427-43.
7. DREAM (Diabetes REduction Assessment with ramipril and rosiglitazone Medication) Trial Investigators, Gerstein HC, Yusuf S, Bosch J, Pogue J, Sheridan P, et al. Effect of rosiglitazone on the frequency of diabetes in patients with impaired glucose tolerance or impaired fasting glucose: a randomised controlled trial. Lancet. 2006;368:1096-105.
8. Defronzo RA, Banerji M, Bray GA, Buchanan TA, Clement S, Henry RR, et al. Actos Now for the prevention of diabetes (ACT NOW) study. BMC Endocr Disord. 2009;9:17.
9. Sanyal AJ, Chalasani N, Kowdley KV, McCullough A, Diehl AM, Bass NM, et al. Pioglitazone, vitamin E, or placebo for nonalcoholic steatohepatitis. N Engl J Med. 2010;362:1675-85.
10. Geng DF, Jin DM, Wu W, Wang Z, Wang JF. Effect of thiazolidinediones on in-stent restenosis in patients after coronary stenting: a meta-analysis of randomized controlled trials. Atherosclerosis. 2009;202:521-8.
11. Nishio K, Kobayashi Y. Different effects of thiazolidinediones on target vessel revascularization with bare metal stents: a meta-analysis. Cardiovasc Revasc Med. 2010;11:227-31.
12. Yki-Järvinen H. Thiazolidinediones. N Engl J Med. 2004;351:1106-18.

13. Singh S, Loke YK, Furberg CD. Long-term risk of cardiovascular events with rosiglitazone: a meta-analysis. JAMA. 2007;298:1189-95.
14. Nissen SE, Wolski K. Rosiglitazone revisited: an updated meta-analysis of risk for myocardial infarction and cardiovascular mortality. Arch Intern Med. 2010;170:1191-201.
15. Home PD, Pocock SJ, Beck-Nielsen H, Curtis PS, Gomis R, Hanefeld M, et al. Rosiglitazone evaluated for cardiovascular outcomes in oral agent combination therapy for type 2 diabetes (RECORD): a multicentre, randomised, open-label trial. Lancet. 2009;373:2125-35.
16. BARI 2D Study Group, Frye RL, August P, Brooks MM, Hardison RM, Kelsey SF, et al. A randomized trial of therapies for type 2 diabetes and coronary artery disease. N Engl J Med. 2009;360:2503-15.
17. Lincoff AM, Wolski K, Nicholls SJ, Nissen SE. Pioglitazone and risk of cardiovascular events in patients with type 2 diabetes mellitus: a meta-analysis of randomized trials. JAMA. 2007;298:1180-8.
18. Dormandy JA, Charbonnel B, Eckland DJ, Erdmann E, Massi-Benedetti M, Moules IK, et al. Secondary prevention of macrovascular events in patients with type 2 diabetes in the PROactive Study (PROspective pioglitAzone Clinical Trial In macroVascular Events): a randomised controlled trial. Lancet. 2005;366:1279-89.
19. Guan YF, Hao C, Cha DR, Rao R, Lu W, Kohan DE, et al. Thiazolidinediones expand body fluid volume through PPARgamma stimulation of ENaC-mediated renal salt absorption. Nat Med. 2005;11:861-6.
20. Singh S, Loke YK, Furberg CD. Thiazolidinediones and heart failure: a teleo-analysis. Diabetes Care. 2007;30:2148-53.
21. King A, Armstrong D, Chinnapongse S. Clinical observations of weight gain associated with pioglitazone: 3 years. Diabetes. 2003;52:A123.
22. Bogacka I, Xie H, Bray GA, Smith SR. The effect of pioglitazone on peroxisome proliferator-activated receptor-gamma target genes related to lipid storage in vivo. Diabetes Care. 2004;27:1660-7.
23. Myers MG, Burant CF. PPAR-γ action: It's all in your head. Nat Med. 2011;17:544-5.
24. Grey A. Skeletal consequences of thiazolidinedione therapy. Osteoporos Int. 2008;19:129-37.
25. Schwartz AV, Sellmeyer DE, Vittinghoff E, Palermo L, Lecka-Czernik B, Feingold KR, et al. Thiazolidinedione use and bone loss in older diabetic adults. J Clin Endocrinol Metab. 2006;91:3349-54.
26. Grey A, Bolland M, Gamble G, Wattie D, Horne A, Davidson J, et al. The peroxisome proliferator-activated receptor-gamma agonist rosiglitazone decreases bone formation and bone mineral density in healthy postmenopausal women: a randomized, controlled trial. J Clin Endocrinol Metab. 2007;92:1305-10.
27. Habib ZA, Havstad SL, Wells K, Divine G, Pladevall M, Williams LK. Thiazolidinedione use and the longitudinal risk of fractures in patients with type 2 diabetes mellitus. J Clin Endocrinol Metab. 2010;95:592-600.
28. Ali AA, Weinstein RS, Stewart SA, Parfitt AM, Manolagas SC, Jilka RL. Rosiglitazone causes bone loss in mice by suppressing osteoblast differentiation and bone formation. Endocrinology. 2005;146:1226-35.
29. Rzonca SO, Suva LJ, Gaddy D, Montague DC, Lecka-Czernik B. Bone is a target for the antidiabetic compound rosiglitazone. Endocrinology. 2004;145:401-6.
30. Lewis JD, Ferrara A, Peng T, Hedderson M, Bilker WB, Quesenberry CP, et al. Risk of bladder cancer among diabetic patients treated with pioglitazone: interim report of a longitudinal cohort study. Diabetes Care. 2011;34:916-22.
31. Neumann A, Weill A, Ricordeau P, Fagot JP, Alla F, Allemand H. Pioglitazone and risk of bladder cancer among diabetic patients in France: a population-based cohort study. Diabetologia. 2012;55:1953-962.
32. Azoulay L, Yin H, Filion KB, Assayag J, Majdan A, Pollak MN, et al. The use of pioglitazone and the risk of bladder cancer in people with type 2 diabetes: nested case–control study. BMJ. 2012;344:e3645.

33. Colmers IN, Bowker SL, Majumdar SR, Johnson JA. Use of thiazolidinediones and the risk of bladder cancer among people with type 2 diabetes: a meta-analysis. CMAJ. 2012;184:E675-83.
34. Ferwana M, Firwana B, Hasan R, Al-Mallah MH, Kim S, Montori VM, et al. Pioglitazone and risk of bladder cancer: a meta-analysis of controlled studies. Diabet Med. 2013;30:1026-32.
35. Tuccori M, Filion KB, Yin H, Yu OH, Platt RW, Azoulay L. Pioglitazone use and risk of bladder cancer: population based cohort study. BMJ. 2016;352:i1541.
36. Filipova E, Uzunova K, Kalinov K, Vekov T. Pioglitazone and the Risk of Bladder Cancer: A Meta-Analysis. Diabetes Ther. 2017;8:705-26.
37. Galli A, Ceni E, Mello T, Polvani S, Tarocchi M, Buccoliero F, et al. Thiazolidinediones inhibit hepatocarcinogenesis in hepatitis B virus-transgenic mice by peroxisome proliferator-activated receptor gamma-independent regulation of nucleophosmin. Hepatology. 2010;52:493-505.
38. Suzuki S, Arnold LL, Pennington KL, Kakiuchi-Kiyota S, Wei M, Wanibuchi H, et al. Effects of pioglitazone, a peroxisome proliferator-activated receptor gamma agonist, on the urine and urothelium of the rat. Toxicol Sci. 2010;113:349-57.
39. Lebovitz HE, Kreider M, Freed MI. Evaluation of liver function in type 2 diabetic patients during clinical trials: evidence that rosiglitazone does not cause hepatic dysfunction. Diabetes Care. 2002;25:815-21.
40. Tolman KG, Freston JW, Kupfer S, Perez A. Liver safety in patients with type 2 diabetes treated with pioglitazone: results from a 3-year, randomized, comparator-controlled study in the US. Drug Saf. 2009;32:787-800.
41. Floyd JS, Barbehenn E, Lurie P, Wolfe SM. Case series of liver failure associated with rosiglitazone and pioglitazone. Pharmacoepidemiol Drug Saf. 2009;18:1238-43.

8

CHAPTER

Drugs Targeting Renal Excretion of Glucose: Sodium-glucose Cotransporter-2 Inhibitors

Jacob Moe

INTRODUCTION

The latest generation of antihyperglycemic agents approved for the treatment of type 2 diabetes mellitus (T2DM) act through inhibition of sodium-glucose cotransporter-2 (SGLT-2), a protein located in the proximal renal tubule responsible for glucose reabsorption. The SGLT-2 inhibitors reduce glucose by blocking renal glucose reabsorption and by lowering the threshold at which glucosuria typically occurs. These drugs have shown additional benefits including blood pressure reduction and weight loss, perhaps via the osmotic diuresis they produce. There is also data to support renal protection and one member of the drug class was recently approved for reducing the risk of cardiovascular (CV) death in a high-risk subset of patients with diabetes.

Sodium-glucose cotransporter-2 inhibitors mimic the chemical structure and function of phlorizin, a compound isolated in the 1830s from the bark of apple trees initially used as an antipyretic. It was later discovered that higher doses of phlorizin cause glucosuria, though its potential for use in diabetes mellitus was not fully recognized until approximately 150 years after its discovery. Interest in its use in the clinical setting piqued with the discovery and characterization of the genetic syndrome familial renal glucosuria (FRG). Both phlorizin and FRG promote renal glucose loss by disabling SGLT-2, either by competitive inhibition or malformation of the protein, respectively. The finding of near normal serum glucose and no significant long-term renal dysfunction in these patients led to a focus on pharmacologic agents directed specifically at SGLT-2.

Currently, there are four SGLT-2 inhibitors approved by the United States Food and Drug Administration (USFDA) for the treatment of T2DM: (1) Canagliflozin, (2) Dapagliflozin, (3) Empagliflozin, and (4) Ertugliflozin. A number of studies have described the overall efficacy, safety, and side effects of this drug class as monotherapy and in conjunction with other agents. Their insulin-independent mechanism of glycemic control provides an alternative to current therapies and may help in certain patient populations where other agents are contraindicated.

BACKGROUND

The SGLTs function by actively transporting glucose into the cell against its concentration gradient. The energy required for this transfer is generated from the electrochemical gradient produced by the cotransport of sodium. SGLTs are large proteins containing multiple transmembrane domains.[1,2] The majority of SGLTs are concentrated in two areas, the intestinal lumen [sodium-glucose cotransporter-1 (SGLT-1)] and proximal renal tubules (SGLT-2 and to a lesser extent SGLT-1). At least seven members of the SGLT family have been identified, but isoforms 1 and 2 are the most thoroughly characterized.[3-5] SGLT-1 has also been isolated in the kidneys, heart, and skeletal muscle at much lower concentrations.[4] Definitive identification of this protein family came from studies by Wright and Peerce in the 1980s after isolating SGLT-1 from the intestinal brush border membranes of rabbits.[3] SGLT-1 has also been isolated in the kidneys, heart, and skeletal muscle at much lower concentrations.[4] Wells et al. later cloned a segment of complementary deoxyribonucleic acid (cDNA) from the human kidney which encodes a protein with approximately 59% homology to SGLT-1. The protein has a similar number and arrangement of transmembrane domains and was thus termed SGLT-2.[2,6]

The kidneys' role in glucose homeostasis is multifaceted, including glucose production via renal gluconeogenesis, its utilization within, and by glucose reabsorption from the glomerular filtrate back into the plasma.[5,7] Renal gluconeogenesis provides anywhere from 20–25% of the glucose released into circulation during the fasting state. The greater contribution from the kidneys to glucose homeostasis comes from tubular reabsorption.[8]

Claude Bernard first described the concept of the renal threshold in 1877 by noting that glucosuria was a product of elevated blood glucose and, more specifically, that this occurred once serum glucose reached a specific concentration. Ni and Rehberg later showed that the amount of glucose reabsorbed in the renal tubule increases with rising serum glucose concentration until a specific limit is reached. When the concentration of glucose exceeds the limit, the kidneys are able to reabsorb and the remainder is spilled into the urine.[9]

More than 90% of the glucose filtered by the renal glomeruli daily is reabsorbed in the S1 and S2 segments of the proximal convoluted tubule (PCT) via SGLT-2. The remaining 10% of filtered glucose is reabsorbed downstream by SGLT-1, located in the straight S3 segment of the PCT.[2,3,10,11] In healthy individuals, essentially all glucose filtered through the kidneys is reabsorbed by these transporters. In these subjects, urinary glucose excretion, the difference between filtered glucose and that which is reabsorbed, is at or near zero.[2,8] In patients with diabetes or chronic hyperglycemic states, glucose reabsorption is actually enhanced and its excretion reduced, further potentiating hyperglycemia.[12,13] The amount of reabsorption increases with rising plasma glucose until a transport maximum (T_{max}) is reached. There is a paradoxical increase in the T_{max} in subjects with diabetes mellitus.[8,12,13] To study the T_{max} in human subjects with diabetes, Rahmoune and colleagues cultured human proximal renal tubular cells which demonstrated an upregulation of both expression and function of SGLT-2.[14] The renal glucose threshold previously described by Bernard is now known to be a function of SGLT. Urinary glucose excretion occurs when SGLT capacity becomes saturated; this is estimated to occur at blood glucose levels of 200–250 mg/dL.[15] The exact threshold differs from the theoretical threshold for both reabsorption and excretion. One explanation for this difference is physiologic variance in glucose handling abilities of individual nephrons.[12]

In the latter part of the 19th century, diabetes mellitus was considered a structural disease of the kidney, the hallmarks of which were polyuria and the persistent excretion of glucose in the urine. During this time, the German physician Josef von Mering found that chronic administration of phlorizin, a compound first isolated from the bark of apple trees, produced polyuria and weight loss in addition to glucosuria, mimicking diabetes mellitus in humans.[16] Animal models have shown phlorizin to be effective in lowering both fasting and postprandial glucose concentrations, increasing peripheral insulin sensitivity, and improving insulin secretion.[17] The use of phlorizin was limited until the late 1970s and early 1980s when the renal transporters responsible for glucose uptake/utilization were discovered and further characterized in humans. Studies eventually proved phlorizin to be a naturally occurring high-affinity competitive inhibitor of both SGLT-1 and SGLT-2.[15] Due to poor oral bioavailability as a result of being broken down by beta-glucosidase, a higher affinity for SGLT-1 over SGLT-2, and significant gastrointestinal side effects, there is significant limitation to the use of phlorizin in clinical practice.[2,11,16]

Familial renal glucosuria (FRG) is a rare disorder in which loss-of-function mutations of the gene encoding SGLT-2 lead to benign glucosuria. Renal function and blood glucose levels remain normal despite significant urinary glucose loss. Heterozygotes have mild glucosuria (<10 g/day) while homozygosity causes severe glucosuria (>10 g/day). Symptoms of this disorder typically include polyuria, enuresis, and sometimes growth/maturation delay. Only in severe cases, dehydration and ketosis (during pregnancy and starvation) or severe urinary tract infection (UTI) occur.[18,19] The benign nature of FRG and the encouraging results from studies on phlorizin stimulated research into SGLT-2 inhibition as a novel treatment modality in T2DM.[18]

The first oral phlorizin derivative, T-1095, was produced in Japan in the late 1990s. This prodrug was created by adding a methyl carbonate group to phlorizin to prevent its degradation by glucosidase, thus increasing its bioavailability. In vitro studies showed a 30-fold specificity to human SGLT-2 compared to SGLT-1; therefore, the major antihyperglycemic action of this compound came from glycosuria via SGLT-2 inhibition. Chronic treatment with T-1095 reduced serum glucose and glycated hemoglobin (HbA1c) levels, lowered insulin and triglyceride levels, and inhibited hepatic gluconeogenesis. Later reported were positive renal effects including delayed development of microalbuminuria, restoration of normal kidney weight, epithelial vacuolation, and normalization of GLUT-2 levels in the kidney.[16,20] T-1095 was not developed further, but the positive outcomes laid the groundwork for the development of more potent and specific inhibitors of SGLT-2. Remogliflozin and sergliflozin are two agents developed with a much higher selectivity for SGLT-2. Remogliflozin showed promise in rat and mice studies with its effect on lowering both fasting blood glucose levels as well as HbA1c concentrations, but it never reached clinical trials. Sergliflozin, on the other hand, progressed to early clinical trials, but this was short lived. The reason these agents were not further developed is not completely clear, but it appears to be related to their pharmacokinetic shortcomings, including suboptimal bioavailability and short half-lives due to susceptibility to hydrolysis.[8,15] In the past several years, more selective SGLT-2 inhibitors have been developed and approved for the treatment of T2DM.

UTILIZATION OF SODIUM-GLUCOSE COTRANSPORTER-2 INHIBITORS IN TYPE 2 DIABETES MELLITUS

The SGLT-2 inhibitors are a class of antihyperglycemic medications approved for the treatment of uncontrolled T2DM as an adjunct to diet and exercise.[21-23] They have been studied against placebo as monotherapy and in combination with sulfonylureas (SUs), metformin, SU + metformin, thiazolidinediones, dipeptidyl peptidase-4 (DPP-4) inhibitors, and multiple daily injections of insulin.[24-28] They work through an insulin-independent pathway and are therefore not affected by beta-cell mass, beta-cell function, or insulin resistance, which may prove beneficial in populations in which these are limiting factors in treatment. In fact, there is recent data to support a beneficial effect on beta-cell mass with SGLT-2 inhibitor use, possibly by reducing glucose toxicity and its effect on beta-cell loss.[18] Additionally, the safety of chronic urinary glucose excretion is supported by patients with FRG, some of whom excrete upward of 200 g of glucose per day without developing hypoglycemia. Patients with FRG are essentially asymptomatic, have a normal life expectancy, and do not develop renal insufficiency or renal tubular dysfunction.[8]

Whereas healthy nondiabetic patients develop glucosuria around a serum glucose of 180 mg/dL, patients with diabetes do not experience this until blood sugars rise to around 240 mg/dL. Studies reveal a decrease in this threshold to around 80–90 mg/dL with the use of SGLT-2 inhibitors.[7,18]

PRODUCT FORMULATIONS

There are six different SGLT-2 inhibitors approved for use in T2DM in the United States, the European Union, and Japan, four of which—canagliflozin, dapagliflozin, empagliflozin, ertugliflozin are approved by the USFDA.[29] Canagliflozin (trade name Invokana; Janssen Pharmaceuticals, Inc.) was made available to practitioners in the US in 2013. Doses of 100 mg and 300 mg are available for once-daily dosing, the 300 mg tablet being utilized in patients requiring additional glycemic control who tolerate 100 mg and have a glomerular filtration rate (GFR) >60 mL/min/1.73 m^2. Canagliflozin is not to be utilized in patients with a GFR <45 mL/min/1.73 m^2. It is broken down by the liver and kidneys, with metabolites being eliminated in feces and to a lesser extent in urine. Empagliflozin (Jardiance; Boehringer Ingelheim Pharmaceuticals, Inc.) and dapagliflozin (Farxiga; AstraZeneca Pharmaceuticals, LP) were approved in 2014. Empagliflozin comes in doses of 10 mg and 25 mg and to be taken by mouth starting at 10 mg once daily. It is not to be utilized in patients with GFR <45 mL/min/1.73 m^2. There is limited metabolism of empagliflozin, with the majority of unused drug being eliminated in the urine (and to a lesser extent in feces). It is recommended that dapagliflozin can be initiated at a dose of 5 mg by mouth once daily and should not be started or continued in patients with GFR <60 mL/min/1.73 m^2. This can be increased to 10 mg by mouth daily in those who require additional glycemic control and have adequate renal function. Dapagliflozin is also metabolized by the liver and kidneys, with majority of eliminated metabolite being found in feces, with a small amount in urine as well.[21-23]

Ertugliflozin was approved by the FDA in December 2017. (trade name STEGLATRO; Merck/Pfizer) available as 5 mg and 15 mg tablets to be taken once daily. Contraindicated in patients with eGFR below 30 mL/min indicated as an adjunct to diet and exercise to improve glycemic control in T2DM. Not indicated in patients with type 1 diabetes mellitus (T1DM) or for the treatment of diabetic ketoacidosis (DKA).

POSITIVE OUTCOMES

Pooled data from numerous trials reviewing SGLT-2 inhibitor monotherapy versus placebo reveal positive effects on serum glucose, blood pressure, body weight, and serum lipids.[29] There is also a growing pool of data to support both renal and CV benefits.

Glycemic Control

Reduction in HbA1c has been shown in studies of all three USFDA-approved SGLT-2 inhibitors, with an average reduction of 0.5–1%. Improvement has been documented in both fasting and postprandial blood glucose levels.[18,21-23]

Body Weight

There has been an observed weight loss with use of SGLT-2 inhibitors on average of 2–3 kg. This is likely to be multifactorial with contributions from urinary calorie loss, diuresis, and visceral fat tissue lipolysis and enhanced lipid metabolism.[18]

Blood Pressure

A reduction in blood pressure has consistently been seen in studies of SGLT-2 inhibitors, both in patients with and without established hypertension. The mechanism of this is thought to be related to osmotic diuresis, natriuresis, and volume reduction. Average reduction in systolic blood pressure is modest, on average 3–6 mm Hg and the effects on diastolic blood pressure are minimal. This blood pressure reduction occurs without significant concomitant increase in heart rate and orthostatic reactions that appear to be rare with use of this class of medication.[18,21-23,30]

Serum Lipids

Sodium-glucose cotransporter-2 inhibitors show a positive impact on lipid profiles of patients with T2DM. High-density lipoprotein (HDL) cholesterol levels were significantly increased in the treatment groups receiving canagliflozin; a small, nonsignificant decrease in triglycerides was also observed in this study. Similarly, dapagliflozin treatment was associated with an increase in HDL cholesterol, however, the difference was not statistically significant.[18,29]

RENAL OUTCOMES

Several studies have focused on SGLT-2 inhibition in patients with chronic kidney disease. As renal function declines, there is a progressive reduction in urinary glucose excretion. Despite this issue, several studies have shown consistent benefit with SGLT-2 inhibitors, even in those with mild-to-moderate renal insufficiency.[31]

Diabetic nephropathy is a risk of uncontrolled diabetes mellitus and once established, the goal is to slow its progression by improving glycemic control. Glomerular hyperfiltration is an early hemodynamic abnormality and is associated with an increase in intraglomerular pressure, which poses a potential risk for the development of nephropathy. This is caused by activation of the renin-angiotensin-aldosterone system and by SGLT-2 and other factors within the renal tubules. Studies of treatment with SGLT-2 inhibitors in T1DM show a positive effect on glomerular hyperfiltration. In patients with T2DM, however, there is a transient reduction in GFR initially with progressive recovery and ultimately stabilization in kidney function, with consistent demonstration of reduced albuminuria. Studies show that inhibition of SGLT-2 and thus reduction of sodium reabsorption lead to vasoconstriction of afferent arterioles (via tubuloglomerular feedback) and a subsequent decrease in this hyperfiltration. There is also a decrease in fibrotic and inflammatory responses in proximal renal tubule cells.[18,31,32] SGLT-2 inhibitor use in associated wiht reduced risk of progression to albuminuria. Small reductions in eGFR are seen shortly after initiating therapy with SGLT-2 inhibitors. However, these reductions are transient and return to baseline after discontinuation.

MACROVASCULAR RISK REDUCTION

Owing in part to the perceived CV risks of thiazolidinediones, the USFDA issued an updated Guidance for Industry statement which required preapproval or postapproval CV safety trials for all drugs used in the treatment of diabetes mellitus.[33] Because of such trials, empagliflozin was recently deemed the first antidiabetic drug shown to reduce CV death in patients with T2DM at high risk for CV events.[34] Clinical trials of canagliflozin and dapagliflozin show similar CV benefits.[35,36]

The EMPA-REG OUTCOME (Empagliflozin, Cardiovascular Outcomes, and Mortality in Type 2 Diabetes Mellitus) trial was a randomized, placebo-controlled, multicenter, multinational, and double-blind trial to assess the effects of once-daily empagliflozin at doses of 10 mg or 25 mg versus placebo on CV events in adults with T2DM and high CV risk against a background of standard care. A total of 7,020 adult patients were randomized and treated for an average of 3.1 years to evaluate a primary composite endpoint of death from CV causes, nonfatal myocardial infarction (MI), or nonfatal stroke. Among the pooled empagliflozin group, 10.5% experienced an adverse event satisfying the primary outcome, compared to a major CV event occurring in 12.1% of patients receiving placebo [$p < 0.001$ for inferiority; $p = 0.04$ for superiority; hazard ratio (HR) 0.86; 95.2% confidence interval (CI) 0.74–0.99]. There was no statistically significant difference in the rate of nonfatal MI or nonfatal stroke between the treatment versus placebo arms; however, the rates of death from CV causes, death from any cause, and hospitalization for heart failure were all lower in the treatment group.[34]

The 4,330 patients trial studying the possible CV benefits of canagliflozin [termed the Canagliflozin Cardiovascular Assessment Study (CANVAS)] completed its 7 years of data collection in February, 2017 with results anticipated later in the year. Expected in June, 2019 is the CREDENCE (Evaluation of the Effects of Canagliflozin on Renal and Cardiovascular Outcomes in Participants with Diabetic Nephropathy) trial. This study plans to look at the possible renal and vascular protective effects of canagliflozin in patients receiving maximum dose of angiotensin-converting enzyme inhibitors (ACEIs) or angiotensin receptor blockers (ARBs). The DECLARE-TIMI 58 (Multicenter Trial to Evaluate the Effect of Dapagliflozin on the Incidence of Cardiovascular Events) will be looking at the CV outcomes during treatment with dapagliflozin based on data collected from >17,000 patients over 6 years; the study's anticipated completion date is in April, 2019. Expected earlier than this is the DEFINE-HF (Dapagliflozin Effect on Symptoms and Biomarkers in Diabetes Patients with Heart Failure) trial, which intends to evaluate patients with T2DM and chronic heart failure with reduced ejection fraction.

Note: This information has been updated in the editorial update 2020.

ADVERSE EVENTS, CONTRAINDICATIONS, AND SIDE EFFECTS

The SGLT-2 inhibitors are well tolerated and most have safety profiles similar to placebo. Genital mycotic infection and UTI are the most commonly reported adverse events, likely a consequence of the increase in urinary glucose concentration. Also reported were volume depletion from the diuretic effect of glycosuria, alterations in serum electrolytes and glucose (more specifically hypoglycemia), ketoacidosis, and bone fracture.[21-23]

All members of the SGLT-2 inhibitor class are contraindicated in patients with previous severe/anaphylactic reactions to the drug class and in severe renal impairment or end-stage renal disease.

Genitourinary Infection

An increased risk for genital infection and UTI compared to placebo has been reported each of the approved SGLT-2 inhibitors. Although not contraindicated in patients who have a history of such infections, strong caution is advised. The majority of patients only experienced a single episode, typically mild in intensity, which was easily managed with antifungal or antimicrobial agents. Across pooled data sources, the incidence was higher in women than men and for mycotic infections than UTIs.[21-23,29]

Hypotension/Volume Depletion

The osmotic diuresis caused by glucosuria poses a risk for the development of hypovolemia and subsequent hypotension, postural dizziness, syncope, and/or dehydration. Events of this nature were reported in dapagliflozin and canagliflozin, particularly in patients prone to such events (e.g., elderly individuals, those taking diuretics, and patients with renal impairment). Patients treated with dapagliflozin experienced volume depletion-related episodes at a greater rate than those receiving placebo. Empagliflozin was not associated with a higher incidence of volume depletion when compared to placebo except at a dose of 25 mg daily in persons aged 75 years or older.[21-23,29]

Hypoglycemia

Based on their insulin-independent mechanism of action, SGTL-2 inhibitors as monotherapy should not produce significant hypoglycemia. The majority of trials looking at the secondary endpoints of hypoglycemia (variably defined) and severe hypoglycemia requiring assistance have found no significant increased risk in patients treated with SGLT-2 inhibitors unless combined with insulin or other agents, particularly insulin secretagogues. Because of this, package inserts of these agents recommend reduction in insulin or sulfonylurea dose at the time of SGLT-2 initiation.[21-23]

Electrolyte Imbalances

Imbalances in potassium and magnesium have been documented among the SGLT-2 inhibitors. Hyperkalemia is listed as a precaution with administration of canagliflozin based on pooled data from 723 patients with moderate renal impairment

(45 mL/min/1.73 m^2 ≤ GFR ≤ 60 mL/min/1.73 m^2).[21] No changes in serum potassium levels were noted in patients with renal impairment being treated with dapagliflozin or empagliflozin.[22,23]

Significant elevations in serum magnesium were also noted in treatment with canagliflozin, both in subjects with normal renal function and with chronic kidney disease. No statistically significant changes in serum magnesium were seen in patients treated with dapagliflozin or empagliflozin.[21-23]

Bone Fractures

An increased risk of bone fractures has been reported in patients taking dapagliflozin with moderate renal impairment and in older patients (aged 55–80 years) taking canagliflozin. The latter prompted inclusion of a warning to consider factors contributing to fracture risk before starting canagliflozin.[21,22] Thus far, there has been no evidence of increased fracture risk in over 12,000 patients treated with empagliflozin compared to placebo.[23] A recent meta-analysis by Ruanpeng et al. found no statistically significant increase in risk of bone fracture in patients treated with SGLT-2 inhibitors when compared to placebo.[37]

Ketoacidosis

One of the most concerning adverse events reported is the risk for developing ketoacidosis with use of SGLT-2 inhibitors. This is often documented in the absence of significant hyperglycemia. Several of the cases reported are controversial or with confounding factors such as severe illness, reduced food or fluid intake, and/or reduced insulin dose. One proposed mechanism involves a reduction in insulin with an elevation in glucagon leading to increased lipolysis and ketogenesis. There is also suggestion of increased renal tubular reabsorption and/or reduced urinary excretion of ketones, based on the latter being observed in studies of phlorizin treatment.[29,38] For this reason, their use in T1DM has not been approved. The underlying pathophysiology driving the development of ketoacidosis appears to be multifactorial and incompletely understood.

- *Amputations*: Orginally reported in CANVAS trial as lower limb toe amputations have not been subsequently reported to be a cause for concern
- *Fournier's gangrene*: 12 cases were reported were identified by the FDA through March 2018. No cases were reported in EMPA-REG OUTCOME and CANVAS. No case was reported with CREDENCE

EDITORIAL UPDATE CARDIOVASCULAR OUTCOMES (2020)

The cardiovascular trials in the past 5 years include:
- EMPA-REG OUTCOME empagliflozin
- CANVAS with canagliflozin
- DECLARE-TIMI 58 with dapagliflozin
- VERTIS CV with ertugliflozin

Study addressing chronic kidney disease included:
- CREDENCE with canagliflozin
- DAPA-CKD with dapagliflozin

Study addressing heart failure with low ejection fraction:
- DAPA-HF with dapagliflozin

While EMPA-REG OUTCOME, CANVAS, DECLARE, TIMI-58 have been shown to beneficial in reducing major cardiovascular events, VERTIS CV trial with ertugliflozin benefits were not clear it was reported as noninferior to placebo.

SGLT-2 inhibitors added to standard care, reduce incidence of cardiovascular mortality, non-fatal myocardial infarction and non-fatal stroke in patients with T2DM who are at high cardiovascular risk.

SGLT-2 inhibitors reduce risk for hospitalization for heart failure and progression to end-stage renal disease in patients with T2DM. This effect is independant of glycemic control.

SGLT-2 inhibitors are now standard preferential treatment after metformin in patients with T2DM and atherosclerotic cardiovascular disease, heart failure or chronic renal disease.

These drugs improve glucose control with limited hypoglycemia risk. Also exert positive effect on body weight, blood pressure, blood uric acid levels and the state of inflammation.

Euglycemic ketoacidosis remains a concerning toxic effect.

Introduction of SGLT-2 inhibitors has had impact as international guidelines. These agents have been placed next to metformin in patients with T2DM and atherosclerotic cardiovascular disease, where heart failure or CKD predominate SGLT-2 inhibitors are preferred choice. The 2019 European Society for Cardiology does not consider metformin as the first line therapy. In those with atherosclerotic cardiovascular disease it recommends starting with SGLT-2 inhibitor.

For details on SGLT-2 therapy, reader is recommended to read as in-depth review just published.[39]

SGLT-2 inhibitors may be of use in fatty liver disease as well.

These agents have been used in conjunction with other glucose lowering agents with favorable results. Fixed dose combinations are available with other oral agents.

Since fixed dose combinations come with different names and dosages, no attempt is made here to provide that information. Healthcare professionals should consult local formularies.

CONCLUSION

Glucosuria has long been considered a surrogate measure for poor control in diabetes mellitus. More recently, however, the concept of promoting urinary glucose excretion has been utilized as a treatment modality in patients with diabetes, marking a major departure in how the disease is viewed and managed.

Sodium-glucose cotransporter-2 inhibitors are the newest class of medications approved by the FDA for the treatment of T2DM. Their mechanism of action involves excretion of glucose in the urine via inhibition of receptors in the proximal renal tubule responsible for glucose reabsorption. Their unique mechanism of action reduces hyperglycemia without directly affecting insulin secretion—they therefore carry a low risk for causing hypoglycemia.

In addition to a reduction in average glycated hemoglobin, SGLT-2 inhibitors offer potential benefits in blood pressure reduction, weight loss, CV risk reduction, and possible renal protection with reduction in albuminuria. The underlying mechanism for renal protection and CV benefits is incompletely understood. Several mechanisms have been hypothesized, including the abovementioned reductions in body weight and blood pressure as well as secondary to diuresis. Substrate utilization and tubuloglomerular feedback activation may also be contributing.

As with all medications, a number of adverse effects have been reported with the use of SGLT-2 inhibitors. Although the most common side effects are genital mycotic and UTIs, which are often easily treatable, there are risks of dehydration, electrolyte disturbances, ketoacidosis without significant hyperglycemia, and hypoglycemia if used in combination with insulin or insulin mimetics.

Studies assessing the efficacy, safety, and effects on CV and renal outcomes of SGLT-2 inhibitors are quite promising, and attempting to further characterize the mechanism of action at the level of the kidney as well as in other systems. Their novel mechanism of action and their effects on more than glycemic control have made SGLT-2 inhibitors a very useful option in the treatment of T2DM.

REFERENCES

1. Hediger MA, Turk E, Pajor AM, Wright EM. Molecular genetics of the human Na+/glucose cotransporter. Klin Wochenschr. 1989;67:843-6.
2. Abdul-Ghani MA, Norton L, Defronzo RA. Role of sodium-glucose cotransporter 2 (SGLT 2) inhibitors in the treatment of type 2 diabetes. Endocr Rev. 2011;32:515-31.
3. Wright EM. Renal Na(+)-glucose cotransporters. Am J Physiol Renal Physiol. 2001;280:F10-8.
4. Heerspink HJ, Perkins BA, Fitchett DH, Husain M, Cherney DZ. Sodium Glucose Cotransporter 2 Inhibitors in the Treatment of Diabetes Mellitus: Cardiovascular and Kidney Effects, Potential Mechanisms, and Clinical Applications. Circulation. 2016;134:752-72.
5. Jung CH, Jang JE, Park JY. A Novel Therapeutic Agent for Type 2 Diabetes Mellitus: SGLT2 Inhibitor. Diabetes Metab J. 2014;38:261-73.
6. Wells RG, Pajor AM, Kanai Y, Turk E, Wright EM, Hediger MA. Cloning of human kidney cDNA with similarity to the sodium-glucose cotransporter. Am J Physiol. 1992;263:F459-65.
7. Nair S, Joseph F, Ewins D, Wilding J, Goenka N. From history to reality: sodium glucose co-transporter 2 inhibitors—a novel therapy for type 2 diabetes mellitus. Pract Diabetes Int. 2010;27:311-6.
8. Chao EC. SGLT-2 Inhibitors: A New Mechanism for Glycemic Control. Clin Diabetes. 2014;32:4-11.
9. Himsworth HP. The relation of glycosuria to glycaemia and the determination of the renal threshold for glucose. Biochem J. 1931;25:1128-46.
10. Kanai Y, Lee WS, You G, Brown D, Hediger MA. The human kidney low affinity Na+/glucose cotransporter SGLT2. Delineation of the major renal reabsorptive mechanism for D-glucose. J Clin Invest. 1994;93:397-404.
11. Jabbour SA, Goldstein BJ. Sodium glucose co-transporter 2 inhibitors: blocking renal tubular reabsorption of glucose to improve glycemic control in patients with diabetes. Int J Clin Pract. 2008;62:1279-84.
12. DeFronzo RA: Banting lecture: From the triumvirate to the ominous octet: a new paradigm for the treatment of type 2 diabetes mellitus. Diabetes. 2009;58:773-95.
13. Farber SJ, Berger EY, Earle DP. Effect of diabetes and insulin of the maximum capacity of the renal tubules to reabsorb glucose. J Clin Invest. 1951;30:125-9.
14. Rahmoune H, Thompson PW, Ward JM, Smith CD, Hong G, Brown J. Glucose transporters in human renal proximal tubular cells isolated from the urine of patients with non-insulin-dependent diabetes. Diabetes. 2005;54:3427-34.
15. Chao EC, Henry RR. SGLT2 inhibition—a novel strategy for diabetes treatment. Nat Rev Drug Discov. 2010;9:551-9.
16. Ehrenkranz JR, Lewis NG, Kahn CR, Roth J. Phlorizin: a review. Diabetes Metab Res Rev. 2005;21:31-8.
17. Rossetti L, Smith D, Shulman GI, Papachristou D, DeFronzo RA. Correction of hyperglycemia with phlorizin normalizes tissue sensitivity to insulin in diabetic rats. J Clin Invest. 1987;79:1510-5.
18. Andrianesis V, Glykofridi S, Doupis J. The renal effects of SGLT2 inhibitors and a mini-review of the literature. Ther Adv Endocrinol Metab. 2016;7:212-28.
19. Scholl-Burgi S, Santer R, Ehrich J. Long-term outcome of renal glycosuria type 0: The original patient and his natural history. Nephrol Dial Transplant. 2004;19:2394-6.
20. Oku A, Ueta K, Arakawa K, Ishihara T, Nawano M, Kuronuma Y, et al. T-1095, an inhibitor of renal Na^{+}-glucose cotransporters, may provide a novel approach to treating diabetes. Diabetes. 1999;48:1794-800.
21. Food and Drug Administration (FDA). (2013). INVOKANA (canagliflozin) tablets, for oral use. [online] Available from https://www.accessdata.fda.gov/drugsatfda_docs/label/2017/204042s018lbl.pdf. [Last accessed February, 2020].

22. Food and Drug Administration (FDA). (2014). FARXIGA® (dapagliflozin) tablets, for oral use. [online] Available from https://www.accessdata.fda.gov/drugsatfda_docs/label/2017/202293s011lbl.pdf. [Last accessed February, 2020].
23. Food and Drug Administration (FDA). (2014). JARDIANCE® (empagliflozin) tablets, for oral use. [online] Available from https://www.accessdata.fda.gov/drugsatfda_docs/label/2016/204629s008lbl.pdf. [Last accessed February, 2020].
24. Häring HU, Merker L, Seewaldt-Becker E, Weimer M, Meinicke T, Broedl UC, et al. Empagliflozin as add-on to metformin in patients with type 2 diabetes: a 24-week, randomized, double-blind, placebo-controlled trial. Diabetes Care. 2014;37:1650-9.
25. Ridderstråle M, Andersen KR, Zeller C, Kim G, Woerle HJ, Broedl UC, et al. Comparison of empagliflozin and glimepiride as add-on to metformin in patients with type 2 diabetes: a 104-week randomized, active-controlled, double-blind, phase 3 trial. Lancet Diabetes Endocrinol. 2014;2:691-700.
26. Rosenstock J, Vico M, Wei L, Salsali A, List JF. Effects of dapagliflozin, an SGLT2 inhibitor, on HbA(1c), body weight, and hypoglycemia risk in patients with type 2 diabetes inadequately controlled on pioglitazone monotherapy. Diabetes Care. 2012;35:1473-8.
27. Rosenstock J, Jelaska A, Frappin G, Salsali A, Kim G, Woerle HJ, et al. Improved glucose control with weight loss, lower insulin doses, and no increased hypoglycemia with empagliflozin added to titrated multiple daily injections of insulin in obese inadequately controlled type 2 diabetes. Diabetes Care. 2014;37:1815-23.
28. DeFronzo RA, Lewin A, Patel S, Liu D, Kaste R, Woerle HJ, et al. Combination of empagliflozin and linagliptin as second-line therapy in subjects with type 2 diabetes inadequately controlled on metformin. Diabetes Care. 2015;38:384-93.
29. Wang Y, Hu X, Liu X, Wang Z. An overview of the effect of sodium glucose cotransporter 2 inhibitor monotherapy on glycemic and other clinical laboratory parameters in type 2 diabetes patients. Ther Clin Risk Manag. 2016;12:1113-31.
30. Reed JW. Impact of sodium-glucose cotransporter 2 inhibitors on blood pressure. Vasc Health Risk Manag. 2016;12:393-405.
31. Scheen AJ. Pharmacokinetics, Pharmacodynamics and Clinical Use of SGLT2 Inhibitors in Patients with Type 2 Diabetes Mellitus and Chronic Kidney Disease. Clin Pharmacokinet. 2015;54:691-708.
32. Fioretto P, Zambon A, Rossato M, Busetto L, Vettor R. SGLT2 Inhibitors and the Diabetic Kidney. Diabetes Care. 2016;39:S165-71.
33. Hiatt WR, Kaul S, Smith RJ. The Cardiovascular Safety of Diabetes Drugs—Insights from the Rosiglitazone Experience. N Engl J Med. 2013;369:1285-7.
34. Zinman B, Wanner C, Lachin JM, Fitchett D, Bluhmki E, Hantel S, et al. Empagliflozin, Cardiovascular Outcomes, and Mortality in Type 2 Diabetes. N Engl J Med. 2015;373(22):2117-28.
35. Davies MJ, Merton K, Vijapurkar U, Yee J, Qiu R. Efficacy and safety of canagliflozin in patients with type 2 diabetes based on history of cardiovascular disease or cardiovascular risk factors: a post hoc analysis of pooled data. Cardiovasc Diabetol. 2017;16:40.
36. Sonesson C, Johansson PA, Johnsson E, Gaause-Nilsson I. Cardiovascular effects of dapagliflozin in patients with type 2 diabetes and different risk categories: a meta-analysis. Cardiovasc Diabetol. 2016;15:37.
37. Ruanpeng D, Ungprasert P, Sangtian J, Harindhanavudhi T. Sodium-Glucose Cotransporter 2 (SGLT2) inhibitors and Fracture Risk in Patients with Type 2 Diabetes Mellitus: A Meta-Analysis. Diabetes Metab Res Rev. 2017;33:e2903.
38. Taylor SI, Blau JE, Rother KI. SGLT2 inhibitors May Predispose to Ketoacidosis. J Clin Endocrinol Metab. 2015;100:2849-52.
39. Scheen AJ. Sodium-glucose cotransporter type 2 inhibitors for the treatment of type 2 diabetes mellitus. Nat Rev Endocrinol. 2020;16(10):556-77.

9

CHAPTER

Use of Insulin, Pumps and Continuous Glucose Monitoring

Aaron B Nelson

INTRODUCTION

In a significant number of diabetic patients, insulin therapy is the cornerstone of clinical management. All type 1 diabetic patients require insulin for survival and many patients with type 2 diabetes mellitus (T2DM) rely on exogenous administration of this hormone to achieve satisfactory glycemic control. Historically, insulin was used in refractory cases where other antihyperglycemic medications and lifestyle changes did not achieve the desired goals. However, randomized controlled trials have demonstrated that implementing a strategy of aggressive glucose lowering early in the course of diabetes can have longstanding, beneficial effects on the development of complications.[1-3] As the most effective glucose-lowering agent, insulin is used both alone and in combination with other antihyperglycemic medications. Insulin has traditionally been injected at varying intervals beneath the skin but with advances in technology new avenues of administration are now possible.

Insulin has been the mainstay of management for both type 1 diabetes mellitus (T1DM) and T2DM since its isolation in 1921. Bovine- and porcine-derived regular insulin was the first to be used clinically and required frequent injections of large doses. The addition of zinc and protamine to form neutral protamine Hagedorn (NPH) insulin in 1946 stabilized the molecule, prolonging its duration of action, and making it possible to combine different insulins into a single injection. Insulin lente and ultralente provided another option for intermediate- and long-acting insulin, but their kinetics proved too unpredictable, leading to their withdrawal from the market. In 1982, recombinant deoxyribonucleic acid (DNA) processing resulted in the development of human insulins, improving purity and eradicating the immunogenic effects of the bovine- and porcine derived compounds. Rapid-acting analogs were first introduced in 1996, followed by long-acting basal analogs in 2000.[4] When injected subcutaneously, regular insulin forms hexamers which gradually dissociate into the bloodstream. The rapidity of this dispersion helps to determine the pharmacokinetics of each insulin formulation. Alterations of the chemical structure of insulin have taken advantage of this, expanding the spectrum of activity from an onset of action as short as 2.5 minutes to a duration of action greater than 40 hours. Concentrations range from 100 units/mL (U100) up to 500 units/mL (U500), allowing for prolonged action and less injected volume for comfort in patients requiring high doses. Differing pharmacokinetics of the diverse types of supplemental insulin make it possible to target both fasting as well as postprandial glucose values.

Many different delivery systems are available, from syringe and vial to prefilled pens with disposable needles to insulin pumps.[5] The pen delivery systems were introduced in 1985 and have been associated with increased accuracy (especially at low doses), patient satisfaction, adherence, and convenience in several studies when compared to vial and syringe.[6] The newer U300 insulin glargine and degludec are available exclusively in prefilled pen form while the rapid-acting analogs, U100 insulin glargine, insulin detemir, regular human insulin, NPH, and premixed formulations (70/30, 75/25) are available in both vials and pens. Insulin lispro, insulin aspart, regular insulin, NPH insulin, and insulin detemir are category B in pregnancy whereas other formulations are either category C or unstudied.[7] Continuous subcutaneous insulin infusion (CSII) is also an alternative that will be discussed in more detail later in this chapter.

Insulin is the preferred therapy for hyperglycemia during hospitalization and acute illness. All forms of insulin are renally metabolized and thus doses often need to be modified in the setting of diminished renal function. The pharmacokinetics of each individual insulin are described in **Table 9.1**. Site of injection, temperature, lipohypertrophy, exercise, tobacco use, and size of the depot can affect the pharmacokinetics of all insulins.[8] Given their mechanism of action, class-wide adverse effects of weight gain, sodium retention, and increased hypoglycemia risk are noted. Reductions in hypoglycemia and more consistent absorption are the major benefits consistently described with the newer insulins.[9-12] It is important to remember that head-to-head trials have not shown any reduction in mortality or cardiovascular risk when comparing the newer insulin analogs to the older, less expensive medications.

REGULAR INSULIN

Regular insulin is the most versatile insulin, available in multiple concentrations as well as routes of administration. The U100 formulation is often used as a less expensive prandial insulin as well as in those with diabetic gastroparesis, to more closely

TABLE 9.1: Insulin activity profiles.

Insulin	Onset of action	Duration of action (hours)	Peak effect (hours)	Concentrations
Short acting				
Aspart (Fiasp)	2.5 min	5–7	1–2	U100
Aspart (NovoLog)	5–15 min	3–4	1	U100
Lispro	5–15 min	3–4	1	U100 and U200
Lispro-aabc	2–10 min	5–7	1–2	U100 and U200
Glulisine	5–15 min	3–4	1	U100
Regular	30 min	6–8	2–4	U100 and U500
Inhaled regular	20 min	2	1	N/A
Long acting				
Neutral protamine Hagedorn (NPH)	1–2 h	12–16	4–8	U100
Glargine	3–4 h	20–24	Peakless	U100
Glargine	6 h	>24	Peakless	U300
Detemir	3–4 h	6–23*	3–9	U100
Degludec	1 h	>40	9	U100 and U200

*Duration of action is dose dependent (approximately 6 h for 0.1 unit/kg and 23 h for >0.8 units/kg).

match their gastric emptying. In hyperglycemic emergencies, such as diabetic ketoacidosis and hyperglycemic hyperosmolar state, intravenous regular insulin is the preferred preparation as its half-life of 10 minutes allows for rapid titration in the critically ill. Regular insulin is also used for the hyperglycemia caused by continuous enteral nutrition. A concentrated form (U500) is often used in patients requiring >200 units of insulin daily, as it requires less volume. This increased concentration changes the pharmacodynamics closer to that of NPH, allowing U500 insulin to both have a prandial as well as a basal impact. It is injected two to three times daily and has also been used in CSII, although it should be noted that the efficacy and safety of U500 insulin delivered by the latter modality has not been determined.[13,14] Prefilled pens have been developed to curtail the confusion of using U100 versus U500 insulin in a syringe.

Regular insulin is also available in an inhaled form for patients who wish to avoid subcutaneous injections. This was first marketed in 2006 (Exubera), but this medication was pulled from the market. The newest formulation (Afrezza) was developed in 2014 and has a kinetic profile similar to the rapid-acting analogs, targeting postprandial hyperglycemia.[15]

Doses are limited to 4, 8, and 12 units at a time. This medication should be avoided in patients with asthma, chronic obstructive pulmonary disease (COPD), and history of lung cancer. Spirometry is required at baseline and at intervals during treatment.

INTERMEDIATE INSULINS

Neutral protamine Hagedorn is primarily used as a basal insulin and is administered one to two times daily. When compared to the newer analogs, this insulin is associated with an increased incidence of hypoglycemia. The use of NPH in the treatment of glucocorticoid-induced hyperglycemia has also been described[16] as has its use in the setting of continuous enteral tube feeds. Insulins aspart and lispro are also available in crystallized forms [neutral protamine aspart (NPA) and neutral protamine lispro (NPL), respectively] that have similar kinetics to NPH. Premixed insulins are also available and can be a more convenient option for patients due to markedly lower cost and twice daily dosing compared to the four injections of basal-bolus therapy.[6] Dosing flexibility is decreased, but accuracy is increased when compared to patient-mixed intermediate- and short-acting insulins. These are available in combinations of 70% NPH insulin/30% regular insulin, 50% NPH/50% regular insulin, 75% NPL/25% insulin lispro, 50% NPL/50% insulin lispro, and 70% NPA/30% insulin aspart.

RAPID-ACTING INSULIN ANALOGS

These insulins are used for mealtime coverage and often make up the "bolus" component of the basal-bolus/multiple daily injection (MDI) regimens. They are also commonly used in CSII.[17] Their quick onset and short duration of action more closely approximate physiologic insulin secretion by the nondiabetic pancreas for postprandial glycemic control. Insulin lispro (Humalog, Admelog) was the first insulin analog to be approved for use in the US in 1996. Switching the proline and the lysine at the 28th and 29th positions, respectively, of the β chain prevents the injected insulin from forming hexamers, allowing for a more rapid onset and a shorter duration of action compared to regular insulin. Insulin aspart (NovoLog) substitutes an aspartate molecule for the proline at the 28th position while insulin glulisine (Apidra) substitutes a glutamic acid and lysine for the lysine and asparagine at the 29th and 3rd amino acid positions of the β chain, respectively.[18] The insulin aspart solution has been modified through the addition of both niacinamide (vitamin B3) to increase the speed of the initial absorption as well as arginine to promote stability. This results in a faster-acting insulin (Fiasp) that is administered within 20 minutes of the start of a meal.[19] Similarly, treprostinil and citrate have been added to the insulin lispro solution [lispro-aabc (Lyumjev)] to increase the speed of absorption, resulting in quicker onset of action.[20]

LONG-ACTING INSULIN ANALOGS

These long-acting insulins have been formulated to make up the "basal" component of MDI regimens. They were developed to provide more consistent, predictable basal coverage for control of fasting blood sugars. When compared to the previous basal option of NPH, these analogs cause less hypoglycemia due to a less pronounced peak effect.[9,21,22] This is especially important overnight in the fasting state. These newer analogs have shown similar glycemic control to NPH insulin, but at much greater cost.

Insulin glargine (Lantus, Basaglar, Semglee) is dissolved in acidic media and precipitates after injection into the neutral subcutaneous tissue. It substitutes a glycine for the asparagine found at the 21st position of the α chain in human insulin and adds two arginine molecules at the C-terminus of the β chain. It can be given in one or two daily injections. Comparative studies have demonstrated that the more concentrated U300 insulin (Toujeo) is associated with less nocturnal hypoglycemia, slightly less weight gain, and equivalent glycated hemoglobin (HbA1c) reduction when compared to its U100 counterpart.[11] Glargine cannot be mixed with other insulins due to its acidic solvent. In comparison to the other insulins, glargine has increased affinity for the insulin-like growth factor-1 (IGF-1) receptor which raised concerns about effects on pregnancy and on cancer risk. Subsequent studies have shown no causal link between glargine and these outcomes.[7,23] A randomized controlled trial demonstrated that glargine had a neutral effect on cardiovascular disease as well as malignancy.[24] Basaglar and Semglee are biosimilar insulin glargine with comparable indications and kinetics to Lantus at slightly decreased cost.

Insulin detemir (Levemir) is bound to albumin in the bloodstream and a fatty acid chain has been added to the amino acid at the 29th position of the β chain while the amino acid at the 30th position has been deleted, resulting in the altered pharmacokinetics. The duration of action is highly variable, especially at lower doses (0.1–0.2 units/kg body weight). When used at doses of 0.4 units/kg of body weight, the mean duration of action is approximately 20 hours. Because of this, detemir is often administered twice daily to ensure 24-hour coverage.[25]

Insulin degludec (Tresiba) forms multihexamers after injection. Insulin monomers are dissociated in a measured fashion, resulting in less variable concentrations in the bloodstream and an increased duration of action (up to 42 h) when compared to other basal insulins.[26] This is associated with less nocturnal hypoglycemia in the clinical setting.[27] The serum concentration of degludec was not significantly different in impaired renal function when compared to normal.[28] Despite this long duration of action and stable pharmacokinetics, this medication is still recommended to be given once daily. Degludec can also be combined with the rapid-acting insulin analogs to form premixed solutions. Both the U100 and U200 formulations of insulin degludec are available only in pen form.

Both degludec and glargine have been incorporated into fixed ratio combinations, blending glucagon-like peptide-1 (GLP-1) receptor agonists with a basal insulin to provide both prandial and basal coverage in a single daily injection. These formulations demonstrated less weight gain and less total injections when compared to MDI.[29] There are currently two preparations available: (1) Lixisenatide with glargine (Soliqua); and (2) Liraglutide with degludec (Xultophy). Each injection provides a dose of both medications at a fixed concentration. Daily doses are titrated as needed to a maximum of 60 units glargine/20 µg lixisenatide or 50 units degludec/1.8 mg liraglutide. Antibodies to lixisenatide have been documented and high titers have been associated with a reduced glycemic response as well as more frequent injection site reactions in a small subset of patients.[30]

INITIATION

There are many different strategies available when introducing insulin into a patient's regimen. When using insulin as an adjunct in T2DM, basal insulin can be instituted in combination with oral antihyperglycemic medications at a starting dose of 0.1–0.2 units/kg. This dose can be adjusted to reach a fasting blood glucose target. If HbA1c remains uncontrolled, a dose of short-acting insulin can be added before the largest meal. For patients with T1DM or those with persistently uncontrolled T2DM, a basal-bolus formulation is recommended. Most commonly, a total daily dose is calculated based on the patient's weight, severity of hyperglycemia, comorbidities, and type of diabetes, generally ranging from 0.4 to 1.0 units/kg. This total dose is divided evenly between a basal insulin (~50%) and prandial insulin, with further division of the prandial dose based on the number of meals (~17% each with breakfast, lunch, and dinner). Therapy can be specifically tailored to each patient based on frequent assessment of blood glucose.[31]

When starting premixed insulin formulations or U500 regular insulin, a similar strategy is employed with 50–66% of the calculated total daily dose given in the morning before breakfast and the remainder administered in the evening before dinner. Premixed insulin regimens have shown no significant difference when compared to basal-bolus regimens in regard to efficacy and hypoglycemia rate.[32] An additional injection of premixed or U500 regular insulin can be added before lunch for those with uncontrolled hyperglycemia, with adjustment as necessary to reach each patient's individualized glycemic goals.[31]

CONTINUOUS SUBCUTANEOUS INSULIN INFUSION

The use of insulin in the pursuit of intensive glycemic control and the benefits it confers is associated with an increased risk of hypoglycemia, which is associated with increased morbidity and mortality. To reduce the risk of these adverse outcomes, technology has been developed to allow for greater dose flexibility, more accurate administration of insulin, and early detection and prevention of hypoglycemia. In addition to MDIs, insulin can also be dispensed through a mechanical external pump. The efficacy of the subcutaneous, portable insulin pump with individualized insulin doses in adolescents with T1DM was demonstrated in 1979.[33] Insulin pumps deliver an uninterrupted infusion of short- or rapid-acting insulin into the subcutaneous tissue. An infusion site is placed (typically on the abdomen, leg, or arm) and a plastic catheter is inserted into the subcutaneous tissue. These devices most commonly utilize rapid-acting analogs for continuous infusion as they have been shown to have less hypoglycemia and superior glycemic control compared to regular human insulin. Of the analogs, lispro and aspart may cause less catheter occlusions in vitro than glulisine[34,35] but this has not been shown to be significant clinically. CSII has been associated with improvement in quality of life when compared to MDI.[36]

Several variations of the insulin pump are available with multiple features in common. All insulin pumps can calculate the amount of insulin to be given based on a glucose value in addition to the grams of carbohydrate consumed. Extended boluses can be administered to closer match the glycemic impact of foods that vary in macronutrient composition. This technology allows for flexibility in dosing not achievable with MDI injection and permits closer matching to patient requirements.[37] Rates can be increased or decreased as needed during different times of the day to prevent anticipated hypo- or hyperglycemia. Temporary rates can also be programmed for planned exercise or during menstruation when insulin sensitivity tends to vary. Patients can administer boluses of insulin with meals or as necessary to correct hyperglycemia. Pumps can deliver as little as 0.025 units of insulin at a time for precision dosing. Some devices allow for suspension of insulin delivery in the setting of continuous glucose monitoring

(CGM)-directed impending hypoglycemia[38] while others can adjust basal rates and deliver corrective boluses in the setting of hyperglycemia.[39] Models can have touchscreen interfaces and can be waterproof. The insulin patch pump adheres to the skin and delivers a constant subcutaneous infusion of insulin. Patch pumps infuse short- or rapid-acting insulins at a constant rate over a 24-hour period. A button on the side allows for administration of a fixed amount of insulin when needed.[40,41] Patch pods are used in conjunction with a personal digital assistant to provide "tubeless" CSII therapy at adjustable doses. "Closed loop" CSII systems that require minimal, if any input from patients, are currently being investigated and hybrids that only require carbohydrate input have recently been approved.[42,43] Delivery methods using both dual hormone therapy (insulin and glucagon) as well as approaches using insulin only are in development.

New insulin pumps can integrate CGM with an insulin pump to make treatment decisions. The sensor wirelessly communicates data to a transmitter, which sends it to the insulin pump. Based on the glucose value, the pump uses an algorithm to adjust the insulin delivery to maintain glucose in target range. In type 1 diabetic patients, sensor augmented pump therapy was demonstrated to reduce HbA1c by 0.6% when compared to MDI.[44] When compared to MDI, use of CSII lowered A1c approximately 0.5% in uncontrolled type 2 diabetic patients.[45]

There are also multiple disadvantages to CSII. Cost can be prohibitive, both when initially obtaining the pump then ongoing when obtaining tubing, reservoirs, and infusion sites. There is also a risk of infection at the insertion site, as the catheter is typically left in place for approximately 72 hours before removal and reinsertion. Interruption of the infusion can occur due to mechanical malfunction of the pump itself or impaired delivery of the insulin due to occlusion of the catheter or tubing. Due to the short duration of action of the insulins that are used in insulin pumps, disruption of this flow can quickly lead to hyperglycemia within a matter of hours. Patients must monitor blood glucose frequently when using these devices to avoid hyperglycemia and ketoacidosis from lack of insulin.[37,46]

GLUCOSE MONITORING

In both T1DM and T2DM, knowledge of the blood glucose levels is vital to achieving adequate glycemic control. Glucose values can be measured in urine and interstitial fluid (ISF), but is most commonly achieved by invasive sampling of blood via fingerstick. Prior to 1970, urinary glucose testing using Benedict's copper-based reagent was the standard of glycemic monitoring.[47] This method was limited as urinary glucose testing only detects glucosuria and could not differentiate between euglycemia, hypoglycemia, or mild hyperglycemia. Blood glucose monitoring followed which allowed for a more accurate assessment of glucose. Early glucometers required up to 50–100 μL of blood and measured glucose by reflectance. Subsequent development of capillary technology allowed for more accurate assessments and required smaller volumes of blood.

The benefit of intensive glucose monitoring and insulin therapy was demonstrated in 1993 and led to more widespread implementation of self-monitoring of blood glucose (SMBG).[3] Both frequent fingersticks and CGM allow for assessment of standard deviation from the mean glucose value, which can provide a more accurate representation of the overall glycemic control of patients. Increased glycemic variability can lead to increased risk of hypo- and hyperglycemia that is not captured by HbA1c values. In many cases, the data recorded on a glucometer can be downloaded and displayed into charts and graphs for review and to aid in making treatment decisions. An association between increased frequency of SMBG and improved HbA1c has been observed in the Type 1 Diabetes Exchange registry. Both MDI and CSII were included in this analysis and regardless of insulin regimen, patients testing three to four times daily had a mean HbA1c of 8.6% compared to 7.6% in those testing 10 or more times daily.[48] Current guidelines recommend tailoring the frequency of testing to the needs of each individual patient.[49] Testing fingersticks very frequently can be both expensive, given the cost of supplies as well as painful and inconvenient for the patient. To address these issues, CGM was developed.

Continuous glucose monitoring measures ISF glucose concentration through the insertion of a subcutaneous plastic catheter. Glucose diffuses into the ISF from the capillaries which provides an estimation of blood glucose. This glucose diffuses through a semipermeable layer along with oxygen and is converted into hydrogen peroxide and gluconic acid via glucose oxidase. Hydrogen peroxide comes into contact with an electrode layer, generating two electrons and an electrical current that is converted into a glucose value. Because of this process, measurements of the ISF glucose can lag up to 15 minutes behind the concentrations in the blood. Values are recorded every 5 minutes resulting in 288 values per day. This large amount of data is then recorded and transmitted to a display system (smartphones in some instances), which can also be integrated into an insulin pump for augmentation. Due to this frequent sampling, trends can be obtained and patients can be notified if glucose is increasing or decreasing too rapidly. Alarms can also be set to alert patients (and their family members) of glucose values above or below their target range. With these alarms, intervention can take place and impending hypo- and hyperglycemia can be avoided. In patients at high risk for extreme glucose values or those with hypoglycemic unawareness, this notification can be critical. As with SMBG glucometers, CGM data can be uploaded into databases that are accessible by patients and their providers for review.

A randomized controlled trial demonstrated no significant difference between mean time spent in target range, hypoglycemia or hyperglycemia in type 1 diabetic patients using CGM only, or CGM plus confirmatory fingerstick monitoring.[50] Previous recommendations were to remove and reinsert a new sensor every 7 days, calibrating the sensor with an SMBG measurement twice daily. However, newer models of CGM are factory calibrated and can be used in place of fingerstick values to make treatment decisions. These monitors have been designed for longer use of 10–14 days per sensor (Freestyle Libre, DexCom), and implantable sensors that can last up to 90 days are now available (Eversense).[51] Noninvasive methods of glucose measurement are under investigation.

Continuous glucose monitoring also has its limitations. Depending on the reagents used for measuring ISF glucose, interference and glycemic discrepancy can occur. Acetaminophen, intravenous vitamin C, red wine, and lisinopril have all been associated with different degrees of variation.[52,53] One study demonstrated that a dose of 1,000 mg acetaminophen (paracetamol) led to CGM values up to >100 mg/dL higher than concurrently measured blood glucose.[54] This risk is attenuated in the newer models. Cost can also be prohibitive as insurance coverage is variable. Adherence of the sensor for multiple consecutive days can be an issue, especially in warm and humid climates. In earlier CGM models, the concordance of ISF glucose and blood glucose was within 15-20%. This difference is magnified at higher blood glucose levels and is also dependent on the rate of change of blood glucose. With advances in technology, the mean absolute relative difference (MARD) in the new models has improved to <10%. Though this change is significant, the accuracy of CGM measurements at low levels of glucose has been questioned.[55] The integration of more accurate glucose monitoring with CSII systems that can make changes in insulin distribution based on the data is currently being studied and implemented.

CONCLUSION

Insulin is a mainstay of management in all forms of diabetes. Modifications of the insulin peptide itself and the incorporation of different molecules into the solution have led to increased dosing flexibility and closer approximation of in vivo insulin kinetics. A variety of insulins as well as methods of administration are now available, but their use must be balanced with evidence for their improved efficacy and increased costs. Frequent monitoring of glucose is key to achieving adequate glycemic control without causing hypoglycemia. CGM can allow for this and can be instrumental in preventing hypoglycemia in those at high risk. Integration of CGM with CSII is being further developed to account for day-to-day changes in insulin requirements and to help minimize glycemic variability.

REFERENCES

1. Intensive blood-glucose control with sulphonylureas or insulin compared with conventional treatment and risk of complications in patients with type 2 diabetes (UKPDS 33). UK Prospective Diabetes Study (UKPDS) Group. Lancet. 1998;352(9131):837-53.
2. Holman RR, Paul SK, Bethel MA, Matthews DR, Neil HA. 10-year follow-up of intensive glucose control in type 2 diabetes. N Engl J Med. 2008;359(15):1577-89.
3. Nathan DM, Genuth S, Lachin J, Cleary P, Crofford O, Davis M, et al. The effect of intensive treatment of diabetes on the development and progression of long-term complications in insulin-dependent diabetes mellitus. N Engl J Med. 1993;329(14):977-86.
4. Greene JA, Riggs KR. Why is there no generic insulin? Historical origins of a modern problem. N Engl J Med. 2015;372(12):1171-5.
5. Selam JL. Evolution of diabetes insulin delivery devices. J Diabetes Sci Technol. 2010;4(3):505-13.
6. Dunbar JM, Madden PM, Gleeson DT, Fiad TM, McKenna TJ. Premixed insulin preparations in pen syringes maintain glycemic control and are preferred by patients. Diabetes Care. 1994;17(8):874-8.
7. Lambert K, Holt RI. The use of insulin analogues in pregnancy. Diabetes Obes Metab. 2013;15(10):888-900.
8. Koivisto VA, Felig P. Effects of leg exercise on insulin absorption in diabetic patients. N Engl J Med. 1978;298(2):79-83.
9. Heinemann L, Linkeschova R, Rave K, Hompesch B, Sedlak MA, Heise T. Time-action profile of the long-acting insulin analog insulin glargine (HOE901) in comparison with those of NPH insulin and placebo. Diabetes Care. 2000;23(5):644-9.
10. Owens DR, Bolli GB. Beyond the era of NPH insulin-long-acting insulin analogs: chemistry, comparative pharmacology, and clinical application. Diabetes Technol Ther. 2008;10(5):333-49.
11. Riddle MC, Bolli GB, Ziemen M, Muehlen-Bartmer I, Bizet F, Home PD. New insulin glargine 300 units/mL versus glargine 100 units/mL in people with type 2 diabetes using basal and mealtime insulin: glucose control and hypoglycemia in a 6-month randomized controlled trial (EDITION 1). Diabetes Care. 2014;37(10):2755-62.
12. Sorli C. New developments in insulin therapy for type 2 diabetes. Am J Med. 2014;127(10):S39-48.
13. Cochran E, Musso C, Gorden P. The use of U-500 in patients with extreme insulin resistance. Diabetes Care. 2005;28(5):1240-4.
14. Ballani P, Tran MT, Navar MD, Davidson MB. Clinical experience with U-500 regular insulin in obese, markedly insulin-resistant type 2 diabetic patients. Diabetes Care. 2006;29(11):2504-5.
15. Chan J, Cheng-Lai A. Inhaled Insulin: A Clinical and Historical Review. Cardiol Rev. 2017;25(3):140-6.
16. Clore J, Thurby-Hay L. Glucocorticoid-induced hyperglycemia. Endocr Pract. 2009;15(5):469-74.
17. Zinman B, Tildesley H, Chiasson JL, Tsui E, Strack T. Insulin lispro in CSII: results of a double-blind crossover study. Diabetes. 1997;46(3):440-50.

18. Hirsch IB. Insulin analogues. N Engl J Med. 2005;352(2):174-83.
19. Food and Drug Administration (FDA). (2017). FIASP® (insulin aspart injection) for subcutaneous or intravenous use. [online] Available from https://www.accessdata.fda.gov/drugsatfda_docs/label/2017/208751s000lbl.pdf. [Last accessed February, 2020].
20. Blevins T, Zhang Q, Frias JP, Jinnouchi H, Chang AM. Randomized double-blind clinical trial comparing Ultra rapid lispro with Lispro in a basal-bolus regimen in patients with type 2 diabetes: PRONTO-T2D. Diabetes Care. 2020 Jun 29.
21. Lepore M, Pampanelli S, Fanelli C, Porcellati F, Bartocci L, Di Vincenzo A, et al. Pharmacokinetics and pharmacodynamics of subcutaneous injection of long-acting human insulin analog glargine, NPH insulin, and ultralente human insulin and continuous subcutaneous infusion of insulin lispro. Diabetes. 2000;49(12):2142-8.
22. Yki-Järvinen HA, Dressler A, Ziemen M. Less nocturnal hypoglycemia and better post-dinner glucose control with bedtime insulin glargine compared with bedtime NPH insulin during insulin combination therapy in type 2 diabetes. Diabetes Care. 2000;23(8):1130-6.
23. Bordeleau L, Yakubovich N, Dagenais GR, Rosenstock J, Probstfield J, Yu PC, et al. The association of basal insulin glargine and/or n-3 fatty acids with incident cancers in patients with dysglycemia. Diabetes Care. 2014;37(5):1360-6.
24. Gerstein HC, Bosch J, Dagenais GR, Díaz R, Jung H, Maggioni AP, et al. Basal insulin and cardiovascular and other outcomes in dysglycemia. N Engl J Med. 2012;367(4):319-28.
25. Plank J, Bodenlenz M, Sinner F, Magnes C, Görzer E, Regittnig W, et al. A double-blind, randomized, dose-response study investigating the pharmacodynamic and pharmacokinetic properties of the long-acting insulin analog detemir. Diabetes Care. 2005;28(5):1107-12.
26. Heise T, Hermanski L, Nosek L, Feldman A, Rasmussen S, Haahr H. Insulin degludec: four times lower pharmacodynamic variability than insulin glargine under steady-state conditions in type 1 diabetes. Diabetes Obes Metab. 2012;14(9):859-64.
27. Garber AJ, King AB, Del Prato S, Sreenan S, Balci MK, Muñoz-Torres M, et al. Insulin degludec, an ultra-longacting basal insulin, versus insulin glargine in basal-bolus treatment with mealtime insulin aspart in type 2 diabetes (BEGIN Basal-Bolus Type 2): a phase 3, randomised, open-label, treat-to-target non-inferiority trial. Lancet. 2012;379(9825):1498-507.
28. Kiss I, Arold G, Roepstorff C, Bøttcher SG, Klim S, Haahr H. Insulin degludec: pharmacokinetics in patients with renal impairment. Clin Pharmacokinet. 2014;53(2):175-83.
29. Eng C, Kramer CK, Zinman B, Retnakaran R. Glucagon-like peptide-1 receptor agonist and basal insulin combination treatment for the management of type 2 diabetes: a systematic review and meta-analysis. Lancet. 2015;384(9961):2228-34.
30. Food and Drug Administration (FDA). (2017). SOLIQUA® (insulin glargine and lixisenatide injection) for subcutaneous use. [online] Available from https://www.accessdata.fda.gov/drugsatfda_docs/label/2017/208673s002lbl.pdf. [Last accessed February, 2020].
31. Inzucchi SE, Bergenstal RM, Buse JB, Diamant M, Ferrannini E, Nauck M, et al. Management of hyperglycemia in type 2 diabetes, 2015: a patient-centered approach: update to a position statement of the American Diabetes Association and the European Association for the Study of Diabetes. Diabetes Care. 2015;38(1):140-9.
32. Giugliano D, Chiodini P, Maiorino MI, Bellastella G, Esposito K. Intensification of insulin therapy with basal-bolus or premixed insulin regimens in type 2 diabetes: a systematic review and meta-analysis of randomized controlled trials. Endocrine. 2016;51(3):417-28.

33. Tamborlane WV, Sherwin RS, Genel M, Felig P. Reduction to normal of plasma glucose in juvenile diabetes by subcutaneous administration of insulin with a portable infusion pump. N Engl J Med. 1979;300(11):573-8.
34. Pozzilli P, Battelino T, Danne T, Hovorka R, Jarosz-Chobot P, Renard E. Continuous subcutaneous insulin infusion in diabetes: patient populations, safety, efficacy, and pharmacoeconomics. Diabetes Metab Res Rev. 2016;32(1):21-39.
35. Kerr D, Wizemann E, Senstius J, Zacho M, Ampudia-Blasco FJ. Stability and performance of rapid-acting insulin analogs used for continuous subcutaneous insulin infusion: a systematic review. J Diabetes Sci Technol. 2013;7(6):1595-606.
36. Hoogma RP, Hammond PJ, Gomis R, Kerr D, Bruttomesso D, Bouter KP, et al. Comparison of the effects of continuous subcutaneous insulin infusion (CSII) and NPH-based multiple daily insulin injections (MDI) on glycaemic control and quality of life: results of the 5-nations trial. Diabet Med. 2006;23(2):141-7.
37. Grunberger G, Abelseth J, Bailey T, Bode B, Handelsman Y, Hellman R, et al. Consensus statement by the American Association of Clinical Endocrinologists/American College of Endocrinology insulin pump management task force. Endocr Pract. 2014;20(5):463-89.
38. Bergenstal RM, Klonoff DC, Garg SK, Bode BW, Meredith M, Slover RH, et al. Threshold-based insulin-pump interruption for reduction of hypoglycemia. N Engl J Med. 2013;369(3):224-32.
39. Brown SA, Kovatchev BP, Raghinaru D, Lum JW, Buckingham BA, Kudva YC, Laffel LM, Levy CJ, Pinsker JE, Wadwa RP, Dassau E. Six-month randomized, multicenter trial of closed-loop control in type 1 diabetes. New England Journal of Medicine. 2019 Oct 31;381(18):1707-17.
40. Rosenfeld C, Bohannon N, Bode B, Kelman A, Mintz S, Schorr A, et al. The V-Go insulin delivery device used in clinical practice: patient perception and retrospective analysis of glycemic control. Endocr Pract. 2012;18(5):660-7.
41. Kapitza C, Fein S, Heinemann L, Schleusener D, Levesque S, Strange P. Basal—Prandial Insulin Delivery in Type 2 Diabetes Mellitus via the V-Go™: A Novel Continuous Subcutaneous Infusion Device. J Diabetes Sci Technol. 2008;2(1):40-6.
42. Phillip M, Battelino T, Atlas E, Kordonouri O, Bratina N, Miller S, et al. Nocturnal glucose control with an artificial pancreas at a diabetes camp. N Engl J Med. 2013;368(9):824-33.
43. Bergenstal RM, Garg S, Weinzimer SA, Buckingham BA, Bode BW, Tamborlane WV, et al. Safety of a hybrid closed-loop insulin delivery system in patients with type 1 diabetes. JAMA. 2016;316(13):1407-8.
44. Bergenstal RM, Tamborlane WV, Ahmann A, Buse JB, Dailey G, Davis SN, et al. Effectiveness of sensor-augmented insulin-pump therapy in type 1 diabetes. N Engl J Med. 2010;363(4):311-20.
45. Reznik Y, Cohen O, Aronson R, Conget I, Runzis S, Castaneda J, et al. Insulin pump treatment compared with multiple daily injections for treatment of type 2 diabetes (OpT2mise): a randomised open-label controlled trial. Lancet. 2014;384(9950):1265-72.
46. American Diabetes Association. Standards of Medical Care in Diabetes—2017. Diabetes Care. 2017;40(Suppl 1):S1-135.
47. Benedict SR. A reagent for the detection of reducing sugars. J Biol Chem. 1909;5(5):485-7.
48. Miller KM, Beck RW, Bergenstal RM, Goland RS, Haller MJ, McGill JB, et al. Evidence of a strong association between frequency of self-monitoring of blood glucose and hemoglobin A1c levels in T1D exchange clinic registry participants. Diabetes Care. 2013;36(7):2009-14.
49. Bailey TS, Grunberger G, Bode BW, Handelsman Y, Hirsch IB, Jovanovič L, et al. American Association of Clinical Endocrinologists and American College of Endocrinology 2016 outpatient glucose monitoring consensus statement. Endocr Pract. 2016;22(2):231-61.

50. Aleppo G, Ruedy KJ, Riddlesworth TD, Kruger DF, Peters AL, Hirsch I, et al. REPLACE-BG: A Randomized Trial Comparing Continuous Glucose Monitoring With and Without Routine Blood Glucose Monitoring in Adults With Well-Controlled Type 1 Diabetes. Diabetes Care. 2017;40(4):538-45.
51. Christiansen MP, Klaff LJ, Brazg R, Chang AR, Levy CJ, Lam D, Denham DS, Atiee G, Bode BW, Walters SJ, Kelley L. A prospective multicenter evaluation of the accuracy of a novel implanted continuous glucose sensor: PRECISE II. Diabetes technology & therapeutics. 2018 Mar 1;20(3):197-206.
52. Vasudevan S, Hirsch IB. Interference of intravenous vitamin C with blood glucose testing. Diabetes Care. 2014;37(5):e93-4.
53. Basu A, Slama MQ, Nicholson WT, Langman L, Peyser T, Carter R, et al. Continuous Glucose Monitor Interference With Commonly Prescribed Medications: A Pilot Study. J Diabetes Sci Technol. 2017;11(5):936-41.
54. Maahs DM, DeSalvo D, Pyle L, Ly T, Messer L, Clinton P, et al. Effect of acetaminophen on CGM glucose in an outpatient setting. Diabetes Care. 2015;38(10):e158-9.
55. Farrell CM, McNeilly AD, Hapca SM, McCrimmon RJ. Real-time Continuous Glucose Monitoring During a Hyperinsulinemic Hypoglycemic Clamp Significantly Underestimates the Degree of Hypoglycemia. Diabetes care.:dc200882.

10

CHAPTER

Chloroquine in the Treatment of Diabetes Mellitus

Beatrice Anne M, Sujoy Ghosh, Sanjay Kalra

INTRODUCTION

Chloroquine, one of the oldest antimalarial drugs still in use, has helped mankind not only to curb the mortality and morbidity associated with malaria, but also many other diseases like rheumatoid arthritis (RA), systemic lupus erythematosus (SLE), and other rheumatological disorders. In recent times, it has again come under the limelight for its potential as an antidiabetic drug. Hydroxychloroquine (HCQ) is an antimalarial agent which resembles chloroquine in structure. It has been studied that the drug has marked effect of lowering glucose levels. Though the drug has been indicated for similar cases, it is not recommended much as it produces very high retinal toxicity. This review article aims to describe this antihyperglycemic effect of HCQ and discusses the future of this drug in the treatment of one of the most prevalent diseases in the world. Currently it is not approved by the FDA for medical management of diabetes mellitus.

GLUCOSE-LOWERING EFFECT

The insulin-sparing and glucose-lowering effect of chloroquine was recognized as early as 1984 when Blazar et al.[1] reported their first case of a diabetic lady with severe insulin resistance treated with chloroquine. Treatment with chloroquine phosphate (500 mg twice a day) had reduced the insulin requirement in this patient from 8,400 to 700 U/day. The insulin-degrading activity, which was thought to contribute to marked insulin resistance, was studied in this patient before and after chloroquine therapy. The authors postulated that chloroquine affects the protease activity (which was responsible for the insulin degradation) in both the subcutaneous adipose tissue and the liver. Smith GD et al.[2] studied influence of chloroquine on insulin and glucose homeostasis in six type 2 diabetes mellitus (T2DM) subjects and juxtaposed the results with normal controls. The influence of chloroquine on glucose homeostasis and plasma insulin and C-peptide concentrations seemed insignificant in normal controls while the type 2 diabetic patients showed considerable rise in plasma insulin concentration through the glucose tolerance test. The C-peptide concentration did not show any significant change in the two groups suggesting that an increased pancreatic insulin output contributing to better glycemic control was unlikely to explain such an increase in insulin levels. The reason for an enhanced glucose tolerance can probably be due to hepatic retention of insulin, attributed to lysosomotropic activity of chloroquine.[3] The researchers previously worked on animals to find the action of chloroquine; they found that chloroquine has a direct effect on insulin-degrading activity[4] due to presence of a class of endocytic vesicle called ligandosome.[5] Insulin gets quickly internalized into this vesicle. Similar findings have been reported in other animal studies as well (**Fig. 10.1**).[6,7]

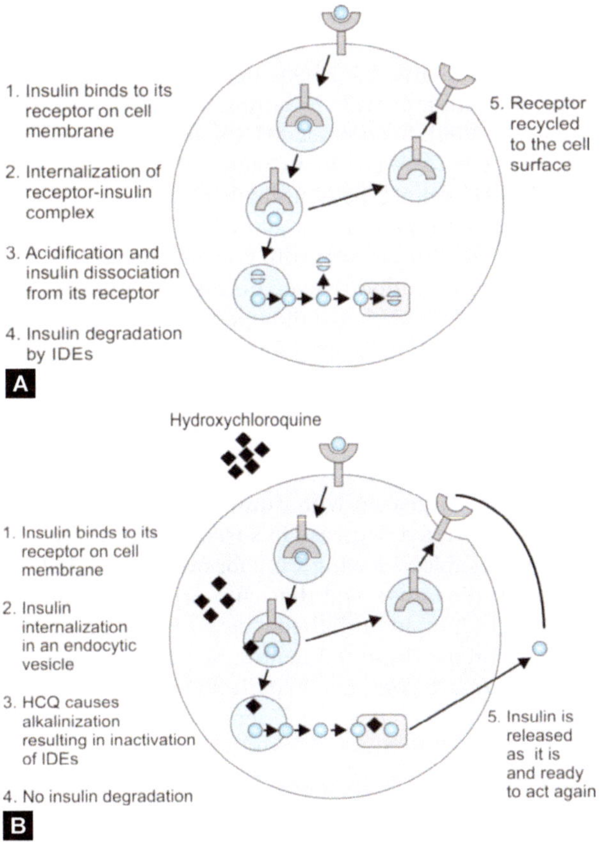

(IDEs: insulin-degrading enzymes)

FIGS. 10.1A AND B: Proposed mechanism of action of hydroxychloroquine (HCQ) in diabetes.

The hypothesis that HCQ improves insulin sensitivity was tested in a pilot intervention study by Mercer et al.[8] The pilot study administered HCQ to nondiabetic obese patients for a period of 6 weeks. The researchers estimated the Matsuda insulin sensitivity index (ISI) and homeostasis model assessment-estimated insulin resistance (HOMA-IR) before and after the treatment. The ISI reported at baseline and 6 weeks post-treatment was 4.5 (2.3–7.8) and 8.9 (3.7–11.4) respectively with a p-value of 0.040. The HOMA-IR also showed a decrease during HCQ treatment, but it was not statistically significant, was attributed to small sample size. There was no significant change in the inflammatory markers in these subjects suggesting a direct action of HCQ in improving insulin sensitivity through reduced insulin degradation rather than through an indirect anti-inflammatory action.

There are studies concerning glucose homeostasis and influence of HCQ in rheumatic patients like those suffering from RA and SLE. Insulin resistance is critical since in such cases as they have increased susceptibility for cardiovascular disease.[9] The activity of HCQ on glycated hemoglobin (HbA1c) was compared with methotrexate (MTX) by Rekedal et al. (they retrospectively studied diabetic adults being treated for rheumatic condition). The HbA1c decreased considerably with the administration of HCQ by almost 0.66% (95% confidence interval 0.26, 1.05). In contrast, MTX administration decreased HbA1c by 0.11% (95% confidence interval 0.18, 0.40; $p = 0.04$). This study had several limitations in that it was nonrandomized, retrospective, and the duration of diabetes in each group was not considered, and patients with concomitant glucocorticoid use were also included. Nevertheless, the findings of this study cannot be ignored as it did open up a new portal for the beneficial actions of HCQ apart from its anti-inflammatory and disease-modifying actions in patients with rheumatic diseases.

A large prospective, multicenter study[10] with a follow-up period of around 20 years reported a lower incidence of diabetes in patients with RA who were on HCQ treatment and this risk reduction increased with duration of exposure to HCQ. The study reported a decrease in susceptibility of diabetes by about 77% in subjects having HCQ for over a period of 4 years or more. Studies observed that chloroquine triggers nitric oxide (NO) in human endothelial cells in vitro[11] and this NO enhances glucose-induced insulin secretion in pancreatic beta-cells.[12] Apart from this, hepatic NO synthase is a part of the production of hepatic insulin sensitizing substance (HISS), which moderates peripheral insulin sensitivity.[13] This effect of chloroquine is also suggested to be a reason to explain enhanced glucose tolerance.

A later clinical report addressed subjects who were not adequetely controlled with glimepiride/gliclazide metformin combination therapy. The antihyperglycemic influence of HCQ was compared to that of pioglitazone. The decrease in mean HbA1c value showed trivial change within the subjects studied; however, there was considerable decrease in total cholesterol and low-density lipoprotein (LDL) values from baseline in those treated with HCQ when elevated values of the same were observed in those taking pioglitazone.[14]

A random, double-blind placebo study was reported by Gerstein HC et al.[15] with the aim of estimating the efficiency, period of activity, and influence on quality-of-life of HCQ and to identify the group of subjects who will react favorably to this drug. The results showed a significant decrease in HbA1c in the HCQ group compared to placebo and this effect was more pronounced in those subjects with a lower HbA1c at the time of study enrollment. This subgroup of patients also had lower LDL cholesterol, total cholesterol, and triglyceride levels after HCQ treatment as compared to the placebo group. HCQ did not have any significant effect on the quality of life. Contrary to the other studies, HCQ was found to have no effect on insulin sensitivity in this study. HCQ was not effective if the baseline HbA1c was ≥13.5%, the possible reasoning being that the patients with higher HbA1c possibly had a higher degree of beta-cell dysfunction and thus may not have responded to any therapy other than exogenous insulin. One more considerable observation in the research was that almost half the patients began to resist the drug following a year of treatment, thereby proving that the existing nature of the disease is unchanged with the intake of HCQ drug.

Diabetes, a chronic inflammatory condition, is characterized by insulin resistance which is related to the discharge of multiple inflammatory cytokines. Chloroquine, as an antirheumatic drug, has been found to inhibit the production of cytokines like interleukin-1 (IL-1), IL-6, and tumor necrosis factor-α (TNF-α). It also inhibits prostaglandin synthesis, leukocyte activation, and leukocyte migration.

LIPID-LOWERING EFFECT

A similar lipid-lowering effect of HCQ was reported in the follow-up study of the Baltimore Lupus Cohort.[16] There are a few proposed mechanisms for this lipid-lowering action of HCQs. Initially, chloroquine hinders production of cholesterol due to its influence on 2,3-oxidosqualene-lanosterol cyclase.[17] Also, chloroquine stops lysosomal activity thereby impeding cholesterol metabolism. Treating cultured human fibroblasts[18] and mouse adrenal cells with chloroquine[19] led to accumulation of cholesteryl esters. Furthermore, chloroquine is also observed to trigger LDL receptor action in cultured fibroblasts apart from elevating the function of 3-hydroxy-3-methylglutaryl coenzyme A (HMG-CoA) reductase.[20]

SAFETY

The retinal damage that could be caused by HCQ due to its usage over an extended period of time is a crucial safety issue. The occurrence of such retinal harm could be limited by prescribing a dosage of <6.5 mg/kg/day on a daily basis as per the guidelines of the American Academy of Ophthalmology. The requirement of yearly screening is currently at baseline and follow-up screening should be once in 5 years of HCQ prescription. Slight corneal alterations have been observed with HCQ therapy.[15] Chloroquine and HCQ causing hypoglycemia in nondiabetics are not a common occurrence as compared to their nonsynthetic counterpart, quinine. Nevertheless, there are case reports of HCQ causing hypoglycemia in nondiabetics.[21,22] Since this hypoglycemic effect of HCQ is dose dependent,[23] clinicians must keep a close watch on blood glucose levels of patients on high-dose HCQs, especially those without concurrent steroid use and patients must be forewarned of this possibility.

CONCLUSION

In conclusion, the multipronged action of HCQ in combination with its relatively good safety profile, affordability, and easy availability of the drug make it an attractive option as an add-on therapy in the treatment of diabetes. Although newer and more effective drugs are available and are under development, long-term adherence to these expensive drugs is a matter of concern, especially in developing countries. Hence, HCQs should be given consideration in this setting and may have a role in treatment of diabetes. Future research should be oriented toward assessing the long-term safety profile, especially the cardiovascular safety and toward determining the minimum effective dose of HCQs for controlling blood glucose levels.

REFERENCES

1. Blazar BR, Whitley CB, Kitabchi AE, Tsai MY, Santiago J, White N, et al. In Vivo Chloroquine-induced Inhibition of Insulin Degradation in a Diabetic Patient with Severe Insulin Resistance. Diabetes. 1984;33:1133-7.
2. Smith GD, Amos TA, Mahler R, Peters TJ. Effect of chloroquine on insulin and glucose homoeostasis in normal subjects and patients with non-insulin-dependent diabetes mellitus. Br Med J. 1987;294:465-7.
3. Dennis PA, Aronson NN. The effects of low temperature and chloroquine on 1251-insulin degradation by the perfused rat liver. Arch Biochem Biophys. 1981;212:170-6.
4. Pease RJ, Smith GD, Peters TJ. Degradation of endocytosed insulin in rat liver is mediated by low density vesicles. Biochem J. 1985;228:137-46.
5. Smith GD, Peters TJ. The localization in rat liver of alkaline phosphodiesterase to a discrete organelle implicated in ligand internalization. Biochem Biophys Acta. 1982;716:24-30.
6. Emami J, Pasutto FM, Mercer JR, Jamali F. Inhibition of insulin metabolism by hydroxychloroquine and its enantiomers in cytosolic fraction of liver homogenates from healthy and diabetic rats. Life Sci. 1999;64:325-35.

7. Garcia-Webb P, Bonser AM. Insulin binding and degradation in isolated hepatocytes from streptozotocin injected rats. Biochem Biophys Res Commun. 1985;128:487-93.
8. Mercer E, Rekedal L, Garg R, Lu B, Massarotti EM, Solomon DH. Hydroxychloroquine improves insulin sensitivity in obese non-diabetic individuals. Arthritis Res Ther. 2012;14:R135.
9. Solomon DH, Karlson EW, Rimm EB, Cannuscio CC, Mandl LA, Manson JE, et al. Cardiovascular morbidity and mortality in women diagnosed with rheumatoid arthritis. Circulation. 2003;107:1303-7.
10. Wasko MC, Hubert HB, Lingala VB, Elliott JR, Luggen ME, Fries JF, et al. Hydroxychloroquine and Risk of Diabetes in Patients With Rheumatoid Arthritis. JAMA. 2007;298:187-93.
11. Ghigo D, Aldieri E, Todde R, Costamagna C, Garbarino G, Pescarmona G, et al. Chloroquine stimulates nitric oxide synthesis in murine, porcine, and human endothelial cells. J Clin Invest. 1998;102:595-605.
12. Smukler SR, Tang L, Wheeler MB, Salapatek AM. Exogenous nitric oxide and endogenous glucose-stimulated beta-cell nitric oxide augment insulin release. Diabetes. 2002;51:3450-60.
13. Guarino MP, Correia NC, Lautt WW, Macedo MP. Insulin sensitivity is mediated by the activation of the ACh/NO/cGMP pathway in rat liver. Am J Physiol Gastrointest Liver Physiol. 2004;287:G527-32.
14. Pareek A, Chandurkar N, Thomas N, Viswanathan V, Deshpande A, Gupta OP, et al. Efficacy and safety of hydroxychloroquine in the treatment of type 2 diabetes mellitus: a double blind, randomized comparison with pioglitazone. Curr Med Res Opin. 2014;30:1257-66.
15. Gerstein HC, Thorpe KE, Taylor DW, Haynes RB. The effectiveness of hydroxychloroquine in patients with type 2 diabetes mellitus who are refractory to sulfonylureas—a randomized trial. Diabetes Res Clin Pract. 2002;55:209-19.
16. Petri M. Hydroxychloroquine use in the Baltimore Lupus Cohort: Effects on lipids, glucose and thrombosis. Lupus. 1996;5(Suppl 1):S16-22.
17. Chen HW, Leonard DA. Chloroquine inhibits cyclization of squalene oxide to lanosterol in mammalian cells. J Biol Chem. 1984;259:8156-62.
18. Goldstein JL, Brown MS. The LDL pathway in human fibroblasts: a receptor-mediated mechanism for the regulation of cholesterol metabolism. Curr Top Cell Regul. 1976;11:147-81.
19. Faust JR, Goldstein JL, Brown MS. Receptor-mediated uptake of low density lipoprotein and utilization of its cholesterol for steroid synthesis in cultured mouse adrenal cells. J Biol Chem. 1977;252:4861-71.
20. Oram JF, Albers JJ, Cheung MC, Bierman EL. The effects of subfractions of high density lipoprotein on cholesterol efflux from cultured fibroblasts. Regulation of low density lipoprotein receptor activity. J Biol Chem. 1981;256:8348-56.
21. Cansu DU, Korkmaz C. Hypoglycaemia induced by hydroxychloroquine in a non-diabetic patient treated for RA. Rheumatology (Oxford). 2008;47:378-9.
22. Winter EM, Schrander-van der Meer A, Eustatia-Rutten C, Janssen M. Hydroxychloroquine as a glucose lowering drug. BMJ Case Rep. 2011; 2011:bcr0620114393.
23. Emami J, Gerstein HC, Pasutto FM, Jamali F. Insulin-sparing effect of hydroxychloroquine in diabetic rats is concentration dependent. Can J Physiol Pharmacol. 1999;77:118-23.

11

CHAPTER

Colesevelam in Type 2 Diabetes Mellitus

Rana Bhattacharjee, Sujoy Ghosh, Sanjay Kalra

INTRODUCTION

As known for years, type 2 diabetes mellitus (T2DM) hyperglycemia is routinely seen in conjunction with hypertension and dyslipidemia. These comorbidities further contributed to microvascular complications like retinopathy, nephropathy, and neuropathy, and macrovascular complications including cardiovascular disease (CVD), stroke, and peripheral arterial disease (PAD). Macrovascular complications are the most important cause of mortality in T2DM patients. Intensive glycemic control has been shown to reduce microvascular complications. However, intensive glycemic control alone has been of less proven benefit in the reduction of macrovascular complications. Multifactorial risk-reducing intervention has been shown to have the mortality benefit in patients with T2DM.[1] This approach includes primarily strict control of hyperglycemia, hypertension, and dyslipidemia.

Currently available drugs for management of the risk factors, particularly hyperglycemia, have limitations particularly in terms of achievement of control and durability of glycemic control. Hence, there is a need for newer treatment options.

Of late, numerous drugs with novel mechanisms of action has been tried for the management of T2DM. Some of them are entirely new therapeutic agent like the sodium-glucose cotransporter-2 (SGLT-2) inhibitors, while others like dopamine agonist, hydroxychloroquine, and colesevelam are drugs which are being repurposed to management of other disease states. In light of new emerging evidence, these repurposed drugs have found a place in the management of diabetes. One such novel newer antidiabetic medication is cholesterol-lowering bile acid sequestering agent, colesevelam hydrochloride.

Cholestyramine and colestipol are well-known first-generation bile acid sequestrants. Recently, the second-generation polymeric sequestrant, colesevelam, has seen the

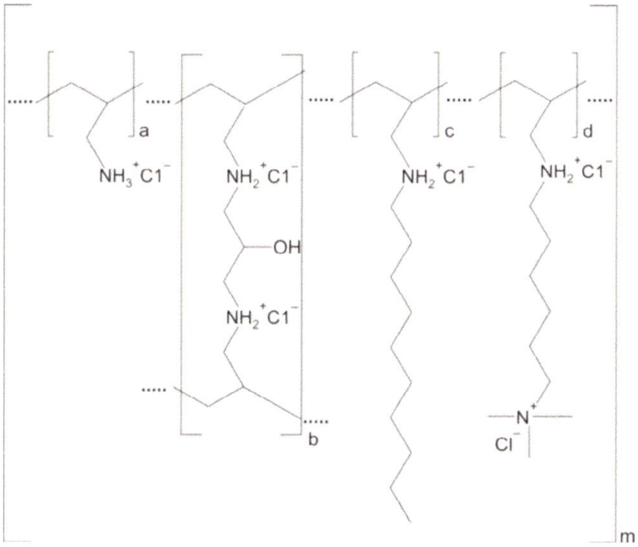

FIG. 11.1: Chemical structure of colesevelam hydrochloride.
Courtesy: Adapted from official product monograph of WelChol.

limelight. It is nonabsorbable in nature and recommended to be taken orally. Colesevelam hydrochloride is poly (allylamine hydrochloride) cross-linked with epichlorohydrin and alkylated with 1-bromodecane and (6-bromohexyl)-trimethylammonium bromide. **Figure 11.1** depicts the structural form of colesevelam.

On oral administration, colesevelam attaches to intestinal bile acids and restricts the enterohepatic circulation of the latter thereby causing exhaustion of bile acid pool. To overcome this reduction in bile pool, hepatic enzyme, cholesterol 7α-hydroxylase, is stimulated to convert cholesterol into bile acids. Further, this leads to elevated need of cholesterol by the liver cells and more low-density lipoprotein (LDL) receptors are expressed on the hepatocyte surface. This is a compensatory mechanism which enhances removal of LDL-cholesterol (LDL-C) from the blood, which consequently causes reduced serum LDL-C values. There might be an elevation or constancy in triglyceride (TG) levels.

The mode of action of colesevelam in enhancing glycemic control is not fully understood. Probably, it might be due to farnesoid X receptor (FXR/bile acid receptor)[2] which is a central regulator of bile acid and lipid metabolism (**Flowchart 11.1**). Apart from regulating bile acids and lipids, FXR seems to play major role in glucose homeostasis at various levels. *FXR*$^{-/-}$ mice have reduced glucose tolerance, impaired insulin sensitivity, and considerably reduced insulin responsiveness in skeletal muscle and liver.[3] Bile acids influence incretin discharge and trigger release of glucagon-like peptide-1 (GLP-1) by way of activating the G-protein-coupled receptor TGR5.[4]

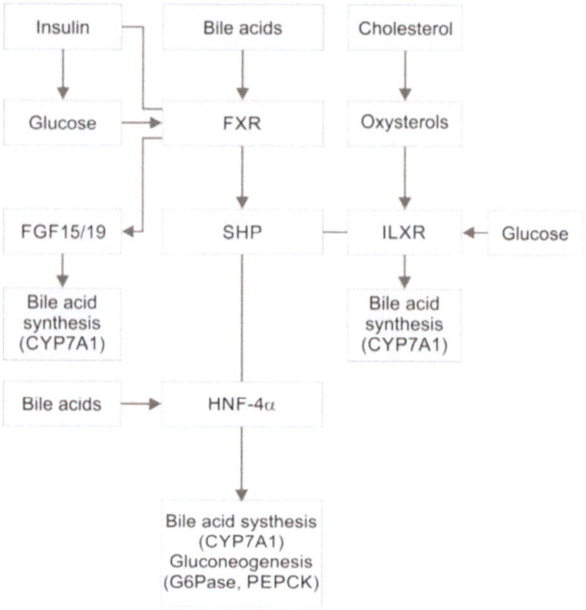

(CYP7A1: cholesterol 7α-hydroxylase; FGF15/19: fibroblast growth factor 15/19; FXR: farnesoid X receptor; G6Pase: glucose 6-phosphatase; HNF-4α: hepatocyte nuclear factor 4α; LXR: liver X receptor; PEPCK: phosphoenolpyruvate carboxykinase; SHP: small heterodimer protein)

FLOWCHART 11.1: Nuclear receptors implicated in bile acid and glucose metabolism.

Source: Adapted from Goldfine AB. Modulating LDL cholesterol and glucose in patients with type 2 diabetes mellitus: targeting the bile acid pathway. Curr Opin Cardiol. 2008;23:502-11.

CLINICAL TRIALS OF USE OF COLESEVELAM IN PATIENTS WITH TYPE 2 DIABETES MELLITUS

Clinical trials have been performed in the United States and Mexico using colesevelam in T2DM patients. In all the studies, colesevelam was used as a part of combination therapy (and not monotherapy) with sulfonylurea, metformin, or insulin.

In Combination with Metformin

A 26-week, randomized, double-blind, placebo-controlled, parallel-group study was conducted at 54 sites in the United States and 2 sites in Mexico to determine the effects of colesevelam hydrochloride in patients with inadequately controlled T2DM [glycated hemoglobin (HbA1c) level, 7.5–9.5%] who were receiving metformin monotherapy or metformin combined with additional oral antidiabetes mellitus drugs. Three hundred sixteen subjects were randomized, 159 received colesevelam hydrochloride 3.75 g/day, and 157 received matching placebo.

As a primary efficacy parameter, Colesevelam lowered the mean HbA1c level compared with placebo at week 26 (–0.54%; $p < 0.001$). Furthermore, colesevelam considerably decreased fasting plasma glucose, total cholesterol (TC), LDL-C, non-HDL-C (–10.3%; $p < 0.001$), and high-sensitivity C-reactive protein (hs-CRP). Triglycerides (Tg), HDL-C, and apolipoprotein A-I levels did not show significant elevation.

In Combination with Sulfonylurea

In a 26-week random, double-blind, placebo-controlled, parallel group, multicenter study was performed. The objective was to determine the efficacy and safety profile of colesevelam in the reduction of HbA1c in 461 T2DM subjects with insufficient glycemic control (HbA1c 7.5–9.5%) on sulfonylurea based therapy. The subjects were on sulfonylurea monotherapy or sulfonylurea combined with other oral antidiabetic drugs. Of the 461 subjects, 230 were administered colesevelam 3.75 g/day and 231 were on placebo. The primary efficiency estimation was mean placebo-corrected change in HbA1c from baseline. Colesevelam lowered the mean HbA1c level compared with placebo (–0.54%; $p < 0.001$). Improvement in lipid parameters was also akin to metformin study.[6]

In another study GLOWS (Glucose-lowering Effect of WelChol study), a 12-week randomized, double-blind pilot study, 3.75 g/day of colesevelam when given to patients on metformin and/or sulfonylurea (who were inadequately controlled HbA1c of at least 8%), resulted in significant reduction of fructosamine, postprandial glucose, LDL-C, and TC.[7]

In Combination with Insulin

A prospective, random, double-blind, placebo-controlled, parallel group trial was performed-over a period of 16 weeks across multiple regions from August, 2004 to December, 2005. The trial was conducted on 287 patients with insufficiently controlled T2DM (HbA1c 7.5–9.5%, mean 8.3) who were on only insulin or insulin combined with oral antidiabetic agents. One hundred and forty seven patients of the 287 were on colesevelam hydrochloride, 3.75 g/day and the remaining 140 were on placebo. The average difference in HbA1c value from baseline till last week was –0.50% when contrasted to that in placebo group (95% confidence interval –0.68 to –0.32%; $p < 0.001$). Lipid parameters were also changed favorably.[8]

The clinical benefits of colesevelam hydrochloride in terms of glycemic benefits and LDL-C lowering seen in clinical trials are summarized in **Figures 11.2A** and **B** and **Table 11.1**.

Ancillary Benefits

The drug in addition to glucose-lowering has been in clinical use for LDL-C lowering. The drug has additionally been shown to be weight neutral, with clinical studies showing a mean change of 0.5 kg (metformin study), 0.01 kg (sulfonylurea), and 0.6 kg (insulin).

INDICATIONS OF USE

Colesevelam is recommended as a supplement to appropriate diet and sufficient exercise to enhance glycemic control in type 2 diabetic adults.

Use in Special Populations

- *Pregnancy*: Pregnancy category B. Enough controlled research not done regarding administering colesevelam to pregnant subjects, though animals tested for this showed no specific damage.
- *Nursing others*: It is not expected to be excreted in human milk.
- *Older population*: No overall difference in response or safety has been reported in patients older than 65 years (or even 75 years) in clinical trials. Nevertheless, elders may probably show increased sensitivity toward the drug.
- *Hepatic impairment*: Hepatic abnormalities do not warrant dosage alteration of colesevelam.
- *Renal impairment*: In clinical studies, colesevelam has been used in mild and moderate renal insufficiency without any change in efficacy. However, there is no data on the use of the drug in severe renal insufficiency (creatinine clearance <30 mL/min).

LIMITATIONS OF USE

The usage of colesevelam has not been sufficiently proved to be administered in type 1 diabetic patients or in children below the age group of 10 years or in girls before menarche. Likewise, the use of the drug as a single therapy for T2DM also has not been sufficiently researched. The same applies to its combined effect with dipeptidyl peptidase-4 inhibitor or its action when prescribed along with thiazolidinediones.

ADVERSE EFFECTS

As this drug has been in clinical use for many years (for management of dyslipidemia) with adequate long-term safety records. Adverse effects were very few and incidence

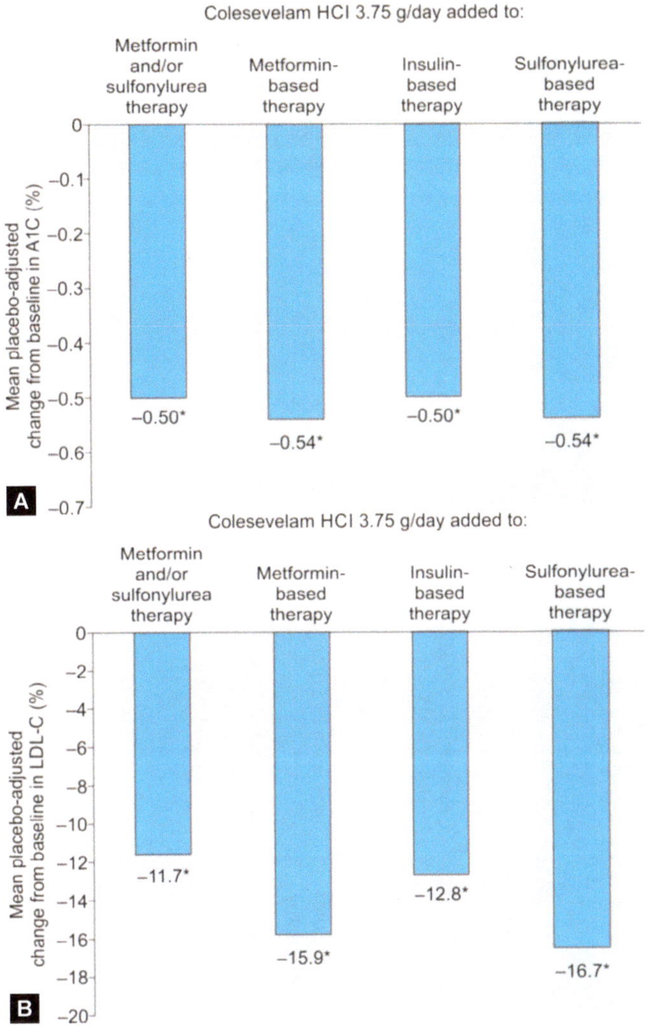

*$p < 0.01$

(HbA1c: glycated hemoglobin; LDL-C: low-density lipoprotein cholesterol)

FIGS. 11.2A AND B: Mean placebo-adjusted change in (A) HbA1c and (B) LDL-C when colesevelam was added to antidiabetic agents in type 2 diabetes mellitus.

Source: Adapted from Goldfine AB. Modulating LDL cholesterol and glucose in patients with type 2 diabetes mellitus: targeting the bile acid pathway. Curr Opin Cardiol. 2008;23:502-11.

of most side effects was not much different from placebo (**Table 11.2**). Compliance with colesevelam was 92.7–93.3% in the double-blinded clinical studies suggesting that colesevelam was well tolerated.[9]

- *Gastrointestinal*: Dyspepsia, nausea, and constipation are the most commonly reported side effects. These are the most common reason for discontinuation of therapy as noted in various studies.

TABLE 11.1: Summary of the clinical effects of colesevelam in patients with type 2 diabetes mellitus.

Studies	n	Duration (weeks)	Background therapy	Treatment	Baseline HbA1c (%)	Treatment difference: HbA1c (%)	Treatment difference: LDL-C (%)
Bays et al.	316	26	Metformin-based therapy	Colesevelam 3.75 g/day (n = 159); placebo (n = 157)	8.1	–0.54†	–15.9†
Fonseca et al.	461	26	Sulfonylurea-based therapy	Colesevelam 3.75 g/day (n = 230); placebo (n = 231)	8.2	–0.54†	–16.7†
Goldberg et al.	287	16	Insulin-based therapy	Colesevelam 3.75 g/day (n = 147); placebo (n = 140)	8.3	–0.50†	–12.8†
Goldfine et al.	509	52	Metformin-, sulfonylurea-, or insulin-based therapy	Colesevelam 3.75 g/day (n = 509)	8.2	–0.3*	Not reported
Rigby et al.	169	16	Metformin monotherapy	Colesevelam 3.75 g/day (n = 57); rosiglitazone 4 mg/day (n = 56); and sitagliptin 100 mg/day (n = 56)	8.1	–0.3*#	–11.6*‡

Treatment difference = Colesevelam – Placebo

*Mean change from baseline

† $p < 0.001$ versus placebo

‡ $p \leq 0.001$ versus baseline

# $p < 0.05$ versus baseline

(HbA1c: glycated hemoglobin LDL-C: low-density lipoprotein cholesterol)

Source: Handelsman Y. Role of bile acid sequestrants in the treatment of type 2 diabetes. Diabetes Care. 2011;34:S244-50.

TABLE 11.2: Summary of adverse effects (AEs) associated with colesevelam in patients with type 2 diabetes mellitus.

Studies	n	Duration (weeks)	Background therapy	Treatment	AEs
Bays et al.	316	26	Metformin-based therapy	Colesevelam 3.75 g/day (n = 159); placebo (n = 157)	• Eight patients receiving colesevelam (four receiving placebo) withdrew because of AEs; of the AEs in the colesevelam group, six were considered drug-related • Constipation was the most common drug-related AE with colesevelam • No weight gain occurred with colesevelam • One patient reported (mild) hypoglycemia with colesevelam
Fonseca et al.	461	26	Sulfonylurea-based therapy	Colesevelam 3.75 g/day (n = 230); placebo (n = 231)	• 18 patients receiving colesevelam (nine receiving placebo) withdrew because of AEs • Constipation was the most common drug-related AE in both treatment groups • No weight gain occurred with colesevelam • Six patients receiving colesevelam (two receiving placebo) reported hypoglycemia
Goldberg et al.	287	16	Insulin-based therapy	Colesevelam 3.75 g/day (n = 147); placebo (n = 140)	• Five patients receiving colesevelam (two receiving placebo) withdrew because of AEs • Constipation, dyspepsia, hypoglycemia, flatulence, and nausea were the most common drug-related AEs with colesevelam • No weight gain occurred with colesevelam • Nine patients receiving colesevelam (11 receiving placebo) reported hypoglycemia
Goldfine et al.	509	52	Metformin-, sulfonylurea-, or insulin-based therapy	Colesevelam 3.75 g/day (n = 509)	• 35 patients receiving colesevelam withdrew because of AEs • Constipation and flatulence were the most common drug-related AEs • No weight gain occurred with colesevelam • 17 patients reported hypoglycemia (one episode of severe hypoglycemia)
Rigby et al.	169	16	Metformin monotherapy	Colesevelam 3.75 g/day (n = 57); rosiglitazone 4 mg/day (n = 56); and sitagliptin 100 mg/day (n = 56)	• Three patients receiving colesevelam withdrew because of AEs • Up to 18 patients receiving colesevelam reported drug-related AEs; the most common were gastrointestinal in nature • No weight gain occurred with colesevelam

Source: Handelsman Y. Role of bile acid sequestrants in the treatment of type 2 diabetes. Diabetes Care. 2011;34:S244-50.

- *Upper respiratory tract*: Incidence of nasopharyngitis and flu-like syndrome was marginally higher than placebo.
- *Neuromuscular*: Myalgia and asthenia were seen in few patients.
- *Hypertriglyceridemia*: In cholesterol-lowering trials, mean rise in TG was 10% which was not significant in comparison to placebo. In diabetic patients, statistically significant rise of TG was noted when it was used in combination of insulin or a sulfonylurea (~20% rise), but not with metformin. Pancreatitis was not observed in any of those patients. However, colesevelam is contraindicated when baseline TG is >500 mg/dL.
- *Hypoglycemia*: It was observed clinically in diabetes patients when colesevelam was combined with other antidiabetic agents by blinded investigators. The occurrence of hypoglycemia was 3.0% in colesevelam administered subjects and the percentage was 2.3 in those consuming placebo. None of the colesevelam treated patients developed severe hypoglycemia.

DRUG INTERACTIONS

Colesevelam leads to reduced absorption of cyclosporine, glibenclamide, levothyroxine, and oral contraceptives. Possible reduction of international normalized ratio (INR) also occurs when the drug was administered concurrently in a warfarin-treated patient. It is recommended that these drugs should be administered 4 hours prior to colesevelam dose.

CONCLUSION

In a patient of T2DM, colesevelam reduces HbA1c, LDL-C, and nonHDL-C thereby helping the patient to achieve glycemic as well as lipid targets. As of recent research, colesevelam usage has been sufficiently proved to be effective with an appropriate safety profile in hypercholesterolemia subjects and as an adjunct agent in uncontrolled T2DM cases who are on single-drug therapy or in combination with metformin, sulfonylureas, or insulin. It still remains under used in clinical practice. It has been approved by the FDA in 2008.

REFERENCES

1. Gaude P, Vedel P, Larsen N, Jensen GV, Parving H, Pedersen O. Multifactorial interventions and cardiovascular disease in patients with type 2 diabetes. N Engl J Med. 2003;348:383-93.
2. Fonseca VA, Handelsman Y, Staels B. Colesevelam lowers glucose and lipid levels in type 2 diabetes: the clinical evidence. Diabetes Obes Metab. 2010;12:384-92.
3. Ma K, Saha PK, Chan L, Moore DD. Farnesoid X receptor is essential for normal glucose homeostasis. J Clin Invest. 2006;116:1102-9.

4. Katsuma S, Hirasawa A, Tsujimoto G. Bile acids promote glucagon-like peptide-1 secretion through TGR5 in a murine enteroendocrine cell line STC-1. Biochem Biophys Res Commun. 2005;329:386-90.
5. Bays HE, Goldberg RB, Truitt KE, Jones MR. Colesevelam hydrochloride therapy in patients with type 2 diabetes mellitus treated with metformin: glucose and lipid effects. Arch Intern Med. 2008;168:1975-83.
6. Fonseca VA, Rosenstock J, Wang AC, Truitt KE, Jones MR. Colesevelam HCl improves glycemic control and reduces LDL cholesterol in patients with inadequately controlled type 2 diabetes on sulfonylurea-based therapy. Diabetes Care. 2008;31:1479-84.
7. Zieve FJ, Kalin MF, Schwartz SL, Jones MR, Bailey WL. Results of the Glucose-lowering effect of WelChol Study (GLOWS): A randomized, double-blind, placebo-controlled pilot study evaluating the effect of colesevelam hydrochloride on glycemic control in subjects with type 2 diabetes. Clin Ther. 2007;29:74-83.
8. Goldberg RB, Fonseca VA, Truitt KE, Jones MR. Efficacy and safety of colesevelam in patients with type 2 diabetes mellitus and inadequate glycemic control receiving insulin-based therapy. Arch Intern Med. 2008;168:1531-40.
9. Goldfine AB, Fonseca VA, Jones MR, Wang AC, Ford DM, Truitt KE. Long-term safety and tolerability of colesevelam HCl in subjects with type 2 diabetes. Horm Metab Res. 2010;42:23-30.

12
CHAPTER

Dopamine-D_2 Receptor Agonists: Bromocriptine in the Management of Type 2 Diabetes Mellitus

Sujoy Ghosh, Andrew Collier

INTRODUCTION

The clinical usage of bromocriptine, originated from an ergot alkaloid, has spanned for a period of 30 years.[1] The agent acts as an agonist at postsynaptic dopamine receptor in addition to being a serotonin modulator.[2] Bromocriptine is recommended in clinics for managing Parkinson's disease due to its functions at dopamine receptors situated at the nigrostriatal tract. The drug has also been used to manage hyperprolactinemia and acromegaly through the tuberoinfundibular pathways.[2]

In 2006, the Food and Drug Administration (FDA), United States approved the formulation of a quick-release (QR) drug of bromocriptine. Clinical studies with these resulted in the FDA approving their usage in type 2 diabetes mellitus (T2DM) cases in May 2009.[3,4] The newly developed FDA guidelines could authenticate the use of a diabetic drug only after its clinical trial showed evidence of no cardiovascular comorbidities. With the new guidelines in place, bromocriptine mesylate was the first drug to get FDA approval as it revealed absence of any cardiovascular susceptibility.[5]

BACKGROUND AND POSSIBLE MECHANISM OF ACTION

The research on the metabolism of migrating birds led to the idea of using bromocriptine in T2DM therapy.[6] Injecting prolactin in photorefractory white-throated sparrow, *Zonotrichia albicollis* resulted in gain in body weight due to increased fat deposits.[7,8] The most important parameter was the time of injecting prolactin, as injecting during migratory season enhanced lipid reserves as proved by the photoperiodically-induced fattening seen in that particular period. Understanding the phases of diurnal rhythms of release of pituitary prolactin is crucial;

this happens in the months of May and August which balance the annual cycle of fat stores.[9-12] With the studies conducted in multiple vertebrates, it has been confirmed that circadian neuroendocrine rhythms have a major role in the growth of fat stores and insulin resistance as the species gets ready for winter season or hibernation.[13] These changes have been shown to be mediated by the interaction between dopaminergic and serotonergic neurotransmitter activity in a circadian manner. The variable body weight and composition according to the seasonal changes are distinct to all vertebrate species, across teleosts to mammals.[14-16] In humans, this circadian cycle and neuroendocrine oscillation are disrupted due to a year-round abundance in food. This results in the absence of a lean phase.[17]

The central nervous system (CNS) partly manages the metabolism of glucose and energy, especially at centers situated in the medial basal hypothalamus.[18] The regulation of hepatic glucose production happens by the sympathetic pathways in the CNS that gather data about fuel availability with the help of its hormones, namely leptin, ghrelin, insulin, glucagon-like peptide-1 (GLP-1), and other signals. The hepatic glucose production and insulin resistance are increased while the pancreatic β-cell activity is defective in obese and diabetic patients as they show abnormal hormonal responses in the signal pathways.[19]

Dopaminergic signals partially control the metabolic pathways of the CNS. Reduced hypothalamic dopaminergic tone is probably related to damaged metabolism, obesity, insulin resistance, and dyslipidemia. The hypothesis may be partially substantiated while taking into account the adverse reactions of agents that hinder dopamine activity like antipsychotic drugs.[20,21] Therefore, it is reasonable to propose that dopamine agonists, including bromocriptine, would have the opposite effect.[22]

The pharmacological activity of bromocriptine occurs mainly through the activation of D_2 receptors, partial 5-HT2B agonism[23] and the inhibition of both D_1 and 5-HT2A receptors.[24] It is believed that bromocriptine enhances glycemic control, averts or reduces insulin resistance, and reduces endogenous hepatic glucose production through creating alteration in the central hypothalamic circadian organization of monoamine neuronal activities.

Numerous studies in animals reveal metabolic enhancements following usage of bromocriptine. The improvements are considerable weight loss, reduced blood glucose and triglyceride parameters, and decreased insulin resistance and enhanced glucose tolerance.[14,25-28] Research in human subjects also revealed identical outcomes; however, the findings are not very detailed.[16,29-33]

PHARMACOKINETICS

Majority of clinical trials in subjects with diabetes[16,29-33] were conducted with the administration of bromocriptine-QR (Cycloset) given as a one-time daily oral dosage during morning; the peak action of the drug happens between 1 and 3 hours after intake. The plasma half-life has been found to be the range of about 15 hours. Most of the circulating bromocriptine (95%) are found to be attached to protein.[34]

The metabolism of bromocriptine happens in the liver with the help of cytochrome P450 3A4 system. Medicines like macrolide antibiotics, protease inhibitors, or antifungal agents hinder this pathway, increasing the circulating levels of bromocriptine. On the contrary, drugs like phenytoin or St John's wort act as inducers and reduce the circulating bromocriptine levels and result in decreased efficiency of treatment.[34]

The excretion of almost all the bromocriptine happens through bile in the feces.[34] A meager 5% of bromocriptine is excreted by the kidneys; the outcome of research studies is anticipated to establish if adjusting the dosage is essential in renal disease. A favorable outcome may be crucial for managing diabetic nephropathy patients.

SAFETY

The relative safety of bromocriptine has been established with information gathered over a period of 30 years from random clinical trials and postmarketing analysis in patients suffering from hyperprolactinemia, Parkinson's disease, and acromegaly.[1,34,35] Adverse effects are quite rare and probably happen with elevated successive dosages. Overall, bromocriptine-QR demonstrated good safety and tolerability. See **Table 12.1** for common side effects. By use of gradual weekly dose titration to patient tolerance, side effects can be minimized.[16,29-33]

Acute adverse events, though infrequent, are psychosis, fibrosis (retroperitoneal, pleural, and cardiac valve), and cardiovascular comorbidities (myocardial infarction and

TABLE 12.1: Incidence of side effects.

Side effects	Incidence (%)
Nausea	26–33
Vomiting	5–8
Dizziness	12–15
Weakness	15
Headache	11–17
Fatigue	14
Constipation	6–11

stroke).[36] When it comes to severe cardiac events, bromocriptine presents considerably less susceptibility than cabergoline, which is also a frequently administered dopaminergic agent.[37-39] The therapeutic dosage of bromocriptine-QR in T2DM is two to three times lower than that used in hyperprolactinoma and 10–20 times lower that that used in Parkinson's disease.[40] To date, there have been no serious adverse events (fibrosis or psychosis) reported in use for T2DM.[29,30,41] However, the potential for fibrosis and/or psychosis in long-term, low-dose usage has not been studied and the effects of cumulative dosage will need to be assessed.[38,39]

PATIENT COMPLIANCE

Despite well-established guidelines for glycemic control, target goals are often missed by patients with diabetes. T2DM therapy include proper following of the recommended drugs, dietary alterations, and lifestyle modifications, all of which play a pivotal role in the treatment. The reasons given by the patients for average or poor consistency in drug intake include lifestyle modification factors like polypharmacy, forgetfulness, comorbid depression, and notions of obesity due to drugs. Adverse effects and hypoglycemia also contribute to nonadherence to prescribed medications.[41,42]

Nevertheless, bromocriptine-QR offers beneficial results when compared to newer and conventional diabetic therapies. Bromocriptine is related to weight loss to a minor extent and shows reduction in severity of hypoglycemia.[16,29-33] Bromocriptine-QR may also lead to slight reduction in systolic blood pressure by about 3–7 mm Hg, helping most of the patients associated comorbid hypertension.[35,36] Further, few researchers claim that administration of dopamine agonists may also offer favorable influence on depression, thus enhancing glycemic control.[43] Furthermore, the once-daily dosing of bromocriptine-QR may fit more easily into daily routines. However, the six-tablet optimal dosing (0.8 mg) achieved after titration may impact adherence.

CLINICAL TRIALS

In the current literature, there are six clinical trials published in peer-reviewed journals investigating bromocriptine therapy in the treatment of patients with obesity and T2DM.[16,29-33] Results from five of these six trials showed that use of bromocriptine-QR leads to moderate improvements in glycemic control and metabolic markers. However, these studies were brief and only enrolled a small number of patients. The brevity is significant, when considering the weekly titration required for optimum compliance and effect.

A research where regular bromocriptine was administered showed absence of clinical advantages as compared to quick-release form of the agent. This proves that the formulation of bromocriptine-QR is crucial.[32] This is consistent with the concept that CNS "fine-tuning" by use of hypothalamic circadian rhythms is important for the improvement of glycemic and metabolic parameters.

There have been two observational trials. The initial trial was conducted in 1992 with a group of 33 nondiabetic, obese patients, and 15 diabetic patients. The group of patients was administered with 2.5 mg of bromocriptine on an everyday basis for a period of 4–8 weeks. Diabetic patients reported lowering fasting glucose, value of which reduced from 15.7 mmol/L (283 mg/dL) to 10.2 mmol/L (184 mg/dL) in those insulin regimen. Those on oral hypoglycemic regimens reduced levels from 12.8 mmol/L (231 mg/dL) to 9.2 mmol/L (166 mg/dL). The mean weight loss in the diabetic group was 1.1 kg.[31]

A second open-label observational study was undertaken in the mid-1990s with 13 obese, nondiabetic female subjects with hyperinsulinemia, who took 4.8 mg of bromocriptine-QR daily for 8 weeks. The levels of glucose, insulin, triglyceride, and concentration of free fatty acids were evaluated from the baseline till completion of the study every hour for one complete day in every subject. Very little, yet important reduction, was observed in the values of ($p < 0.05$) plasma glucose, triglycerides, and free fatty acids. The range of variation in plasma glucose was lesser than 1 mmol/L (18 mg/dL) and this change was noticed in about 3 hours duration postfood intake. The 24-hour insulin level did not show any considerable modification.[29]

Cincotta et al. performed almost four double-blind, placebo-controlled trials with bromocriptine-QR. The first trial involved about a dozen of obese subjects who had impaired glucose tolerance and five obese T2DM patients. About eight of these subjects were given bromocriptine-QR every day in the dose of 1.6–2.4 mg. Follow-up post 18 weeks presented a considerable reduction in body weight in the subjects, the range of weight reduction being 6.3 ± 1.5 kg ($p < 0.01$). The treatment group also showed a 46% reduction in area under the serum glucose curve when an oral glucose tolerance test ($p < 0.02$) was performed in contrast to the baseline.[44]

The next two double-blind, placebo-controlled trials examined the benefit of bromocriptine-QR in overweight T2DM patients who presented with considerable enhancements in metabolic parameters. The initial study was done on 22 subjects and the follow-up of the study extended for a period of 16 weeks. By the completion, fasting plasma glucose reduced by 0.9 mmol/L (17 mg/dL), average variation in plasma glucose following oral glucose tolerance testing became lesser by 1.2 mmol/L (22 mg/dL), and glycated hemoglobin (HbA1c) was reduced by 0.6% in contrast to the placebo group.[16] The next trial had 40 subjects participating and the duration of study was 3 months. There was reduction of fasting plasma glucose by 1.5 mmol/L (27 mg/dL) and improvement of HbA1c by 1.5% (16 mmol/mol) in contrast to the placebo group.[30]

A final double-blind, placebo-controlled trial had 13 overweight diabetic subjects. The regular bromocriptine was administered to the subjects two times every day. The study extended for 6–8 months and the follow-up done after a regular lunch did not show significant variations in percentage of body fat, visceral fat, or in the homeostasis model assessment of insulin resistance.[32]

Two clinical presentations essentially describing different aspects of the same 52-week trial of bromocriptine-QR treatment in T2DM have been presented at the American Diabetes Association (ADA). The first presentation was at the 2008 annual ADA meeting. This study randomized 3,070 diabetic patients to receive either bromocriptine-QR or a placebo at a ratio of 2:1 and in addition to their usual diabetic therapy. The researchers described a decrease in relative susceptibility to cardiovascular comorbidities by about 42% with the intake of bromocriptine-QR ($p = 0.036$; 1.5% bromocriptine-QR vs. 2.96% placebo event rate). Nevertheless, both the treatment group and placebo group reported considerable variation in baseline level, especially the placebo group reporting higher chances of stroke.[45] Another ADA presentation that was conducted in 2009 examined glycemic control markers in the same trial. This demonstration concentrated more on that set of subjects who showed unfavorable outcomes with thiazolidinedione therapy ($n = 56$ bromocriptine-QR group; $n = 68$ placebo group). 1-year follow-up revealed lesser values of HbA1c in the bromocriptine-QR group in contrast to the placebo. Bromocriptine-QR therapy in those who showed a baseline HbA1c of >8.5% or >7.5% resulted in reduced HbA1c by 1.21% ($p < 0.05$) and 0.57% ($p < 0.05$), respectively in contrast to the placebo group.[46]

These group of researchers conducted three more trials using bromocriptine-QR. Over a period of 24 weeks, respectively to manage T2DM, the outcomes were reported online. The initial 24-week trial was conducted on 159 uncontrolled T2DM subjects who were administered either bromocriptine-QR monotherapy or placebo monotherapy. The follow-up post 24 weeks revealed reduction in HbA1c by 0.1% in those who took bromocriptine-QR group (baseline HbA1c = 9.0%) when compared to 0.3% rise in the same parameter in the placebo group ($p < 0.05$). The next 24-week trial, "Study L", was performed on T2DM subjects who were inadequately controlled taking sulfonylurea therapy. About 249 subjects were administered bromocriptine-QR or a placebo along with their existing medication. A follow-up post 24 weeks revealed reduced HbA1c value by 0.4% in the bromocriptine-QR group (baseline HbA1c = 9.0%) when compared to 0.3% elevation in the placebo group ($p < 0.001$). The last 24-week trial, "Study K", was also performed on 245 subjects who were T2DM patients, insufficiently managed by sulfonylurea therapy. The participants were administered either bromocriptine-QR or placebo apart from their existing medication. Follow-up post 24 weeks showed reduced HbA1c by 0.1% in the bromocriptine-QR group (baseline HbA1c = 9.3%) and elevated HbA1c by 0.4% in the placebo group ($p < 0.001$).

The outcomes of the above mentioned four clinical trials became the foundation for the FDA approval of use of bromocriptine-QR for T2DM therapy. The outcome reports of these studies played a major role statistically; yet the meager enhancements observed in diabetic control may not translate into significant clinical impact. The reported reduction in cardiovascular events with the use of bromocriptine-QR can be attributed to reduction in the function of the sympathetic nervous system and renin–angiotensin axis and re-establishment of diurnal changes in the pituitary-adrenal axis. Nevertheless, one more reason could be decreasing insulin resistance that could possibly cause reduction in hepatic glucose production and more uptake of glucose thereby reducing the levels of postprandial glucose, free fatty acids, and triglycerides, which finally lead to reduction in inflammation, oxidative stress, and accumulation of atheroma.[46,47]

Where Now?

Modern agents of therapy for managing T2DM are reassuring a favorable change in the path of disease progression. However, the newer agents are mostly too costly and also offer less favorable safety profile when used over a longer period of time.[48-51] The FDA has approved the administration of bromocriptine-QR "as an adjunct to food and physical exercise to enhance glycemic control in type 2 diabetic adults". The FDA has also added that bromocriptine is not supposed to be recommended to manage type 1 diabetes mellitus (T1DM) or diabetic ketoacidosis.

At present bromocriptine-QR, the drug cannot be assumed as the first-line pharmacological management of T2DM.

To summarize, the potential benefits of bromocriptine-QR are:
- Single daily dose
- Safe use with other diabetic therapies
- Use of circadian rhythms and neuroendocrine pathways in a novel mechanism, separate from current targets of diabetic therapy
- Reduced incidence of cardiovascular events

- Potentially safe in renal impairment, although further research is required.

As of now, the position of bromocriptine-QR in management of patients with T2DM is approved to be given as 0.8 mg in AM that may be increase by 0.8 mg weekly maximum dose of 4.8 mg. It is proposed that bromocriptine should offer optimal influence if prescribed early during course of the disease, may be when combined with other disease-modifying therapeutic agents like metformin, pioglitazone, GLP-1 agonists, or sodium-glucose cotransporter-2 (SGLT-2) inhibitors. Trials involving large group of subjects are required to establish the advantages of bromocriptine-QR for managing T2DM patients and to evaluate result over an extended period of time. it is marketed as cycle set in the USA.

REFERENCES

1. Coloa A, Di Sarno A, Guerra E, De Leo M, Mentone A, Lombardi G. Drug insight: Cabergoline and bromocriptine in the treatment of hyperprolactinemia in men and women. Nat Clin Pract Endocrinol Metab. 2006;2:200-10.
2. Kvernmo T, Hartter S, Burger E. A Review of the Receptor Binding and Pharmacokinetic Properties of Dopamine Agonists. Clin Ther. 2006;28:1065-78.
3. US Food and Drug Administration (USFDA). (2009). Cycloset (bromocriptine mesylate) tablets, oral. [online] Available from http://www.accessdata.fda.gov/drugsatfda_docs/label/2009/020866lbl.pdf. [Last accessed February, 2020].
4. Waknine Y. (2009). FDA Approvals: Fanapt and Cycloset. [online] Available from https://www.medscape.org/viewarticle/702793. [Last accessed February, 2020].
5. Hennessy T. Old Parkinson's Drug Tweaked into Diabetes Treatment. New York: Associated Press; 2009.
6. Meier AH, Farner DS, King JR. A possible endocrine basis for migratory behaviour in the white-crowned sparrow, Zonotrichia leucophrys gambelii. Anim Behav. 1965;13:453-65.
7. Meier AH, Martin D. Temporal synergism of corticosterone and prolactin controlling fat storage in the white-throated sparrow, Zonotrichia albicollis. Gen Comp Endocrinol. 1971;17:311-8.
8. Meier AH, Fivizzani AJ. Changes in the daily rhythms of plasma corticosterone concentration related to seasonal conditions in the white-throated sparrow, Zonotrichia albicollis. Proc Soc Exp Biol Med. 1975;150:356-62.
9. Meier AH, Farner DS. A possible endocrine basis for premigratory fattening in the white-crowned sparrow, Zonotrichia leucophrys gambelii (Nuttall). Gen Comp Endocrinol. 1964;4:584-95.
10. Meier AH, Davis KB. Diurnal variations of the fattening response to prolactin in the white-throated sparrow, Zonotrichia albicollis. Gen Comp Endocrinol. 1967;8:110-4.
11. Young R. Fat, energy and mammalian survival. Am Zool. 1976;16:699-710.
12. Meier AH, Cincotta A. Circadian rhythms regulate the expression of the thrifty genotype/phenotype. Diabetes Rev. 1996;4:464-87.
13. Cincotta A, Schiller B, Landry RJ, Herbert SJ, Miers W, Meier A. Circadian Neuroendocrine role in age-related changes in body fat stores and insulin sensitivity of the male Sprague-Dawley rat. Diabetes Rev. 1996;4: 464-87.
14. Southern LL, Cincotta AH, Meier AH, Bidner TD, Watkins KL. Bromocriptine-induced reduction of body fat in pigs. J Anim Sci. 1990;68:931-6.

15. Pijl H, Ohashi S, Matsuda M, Miyazaki A, Mahankali A, Kumar V, et al. Bromocriptine: a novel approach to the treatment of type 2 diabetes. Diabetes Care. 2000;23:1154-61.
16. Kerr JL, Timpe EM, Petkewicz KA. Bromocriptine mesylate for glycemic control in type 2 diabetes mellitus. Ann Pharmacother. 2010;44:1777-85.
17. Sandoval D, Costa D, Seeley RJ. The integrative role of CNS fuel-sensing mechanisms in energy balance and glucose regulation. Ann Rev Physiol. 2008;70:513-35.
18. Defronzo RA. Banting Lecture. From the triumvirate to the ominous octet: a new paradigm for the treatment of type 2 diabetes mellitus. Diabetes. 2009;58:773-95.
19. Tschoner A, Engl J, Laimer M, Kaser S, Rettenbacher M, Fleischhacker WW, et al. Metabolic side effects of antipsychotic medication. Int J Clin Pract. 2007;61:1356-70.
20. Holt RL, Peveler RC. Obesity, serious mental illness and antipsychotic drugs. Diabetes Obes Metab. 2009;11:665-79.
21. Cincotta AH, Meier AH, Cincotta M. Bromocriptine improves glycaemic control and serum lipid profile in obese type 2 diabetic subjects: A new approach in the treatment of diabetes. Expert Opin Investig Drugs. 1999;8:1683-707.
22. Tan EK, Jankovic J. Choosing dopamine antagonists in Parkinson's disease. Clin Neuropharmacol. 2001;24:247-53.
23. Jahnichen S, Horowski R, Pertz HH. Agonism at 5-HT2B receptors is not a class effect of the ergolines. Eur J Pharmacol. 2005;513:225-8.
24. Cincotta AH, Meier AH. Reductions of body fat stores and total plasma cholesterol and triglyceride concentrations in several species by bromocriptine treatment. Life Sci. 1989;45:2247-54.
25. Cincotta AH, Meier AH, Southern LL. Bromocriptine alters hormone rhythms and lipid metabolism in swine. Ann Nutr Metab. 1989;33:305-14.
26. Cincotta AH, Schiller BC, Meier AH. Bromocriptine inhibits the seasonally occurring obesity, hyperinsulinaemia, insulin resistance, and impaired glucose tolerance in the Syrian hamster, Mesocricetus auratus. Metabolism. 1991;40:639-44.
27. Cincotta AH, MacEachern TA, Meier AH. Bromocriptine redirects the metabolism and prevents seasonal onset of obese hyperinsulinaemic state in Syrian hamsters. Am J Physiol. 1993;264:E285-93.
28. Cincotta AH, Meier AH. Bromocriptine (Ergoset) reduces body weight and improves glucose tolerance in obese subjects. Diabetes Care. 1996;19:667-70.
29. Aminorroaya A, Janghorbani M, Ramezani M, Haghighi S, Amini M. Does bromocriptine improve glycaemic control of obese type-2 diabetes? Horm Res. 2004;62:55-9.
30. Meier AH, Cincotta AH, Lovell WC. Timed bromocriptine administration reduces body fat stores in obese subject and hyperglycemia in type II diabetics. Experientia. 1992;48:248-53.
31. Wasada T, Kawahara R, Iwamoto I. Lack of evidence for bromocriptine effect on glucose tolerance, insulin resistance, and body fat stores in obese type 2 diabetic patients. Diabetes Care. 2000;23:1039-40.
32. Van Hilten JJ, Ramaker CC, Stowe RI, Ives NJ. Bromocriptine versus levodopa in early Parkinson's disease. Cochrane Database Syst Rev. 2007;4:CD002258.
33. Weil C. The safety of bromocriptine in long-term use: a review of the literature. Curr Med Res Opin. 1986;10:25-51.
34. Maurer G, Schreier E, Delaborde S, Nufer R, Shukla AP. Fate and disposition of bromocriptine in animals and man. II: Absorption, Elimination and Metabolism. Eur J Drug Metab Pharmacokinet. 1983;8:51-62.
35. Wiggins J, Skinner C. Bromocriptine induced pleuropulmonary fibrosis. Thorax. 1986;41:328-30.
36. Horvath J, Fross RD, Kleiner-Fisman G, Lerch R, Stalder H, Liaudat S, et al. Severe multivalvular heart disease: a new complication of the ergot derivative dopamine antagonists. Mov Disord. 2004;19:656-62.

37. Zanettini R, Antonini A, Gatto G, Gentile R, Tesei S, Pezzoli G. Valvular heart disease and the use of dopamine agonists for Parkinson's disease. N Engl J Med. 2007;356:39-46.
38. Serratice J, Disdier P, Habib G, Viallet F, Weiller PJ. Fibrotic valvular heart disease subsequent to bromocriptine treatment. Cardiol Rev. 2002;10:334-6.
39. Donnan PT, MacDonald TM, Morris AD. Adherence to the prescribed oral hypoglycaemic medication in a population of patients with type 2 diabetes: a retrospective cohort. Diabet Med. 2002;19:279-84.
40. Daly JM, Hartz AJ, Xu Y, Levy BT, James PA, Merchant ML, et al. An assessment of attitudes, behaviors, and outcomes of patients with type 2 diabetes. J Am Board Fam Med. 2009;22:280-90.
41. Katzenschlager R, Head J, Schrag A, Ben-Shlomo Y, Evans A, Lees AJ. Fourteen-year final report of the randomised PDRG-UK trial comparing three initial treatment in PD. Neurology. 2008;71:474-80.
42. Kok P, Roelfsema F, Frolich M, Van Pelt J, Stokkel MP, Meinders AE, et al. Activation of D2 receptors simultaneously ameliorates various features of obese women. Am J Physiol Endocrinol Metab. 2006;291:E1038-43.
43. Clausius N, Born C, Grunze H. The relevance of dopamine agonists in the treatment of depression. Neuropsychiatry. 2009;23:15-25.
44. Kamath V, Jones CN, Yip JC, Varasteh BB, Cincotta AH, Reaven GM, et al. Effects of a quick-release form of bromocriptine (Ergoset) on fasting and postprandial plasma glucose, insulin, lipid, and lipoprotein concentrations in obese nondiabetic hyperinsulinemic women. Diabetes Care. 1997;20:1697-701.
45. Scranton R, Cincotta A, Gaziano JM. The effect of time Cycloset (a quick release formulation of Bromocriptine mesylate) on cardiovascular events in patients with type 2 diabetes. Diabetes. 2008;57:A95.
46. Bell DS. Why does quick-release bromocriptine decrease cardiac events? Diabetes Obes Metab. 2011;13:880-4.
47. Chamarthi B, Gaziano JM, Blonde L, Vinik A, Scranton RE, Ezrokhi M, et al. Timed Bromocriptine-QR Therapy Reduces Progression of Cardiovascular Disease and Dysglycemia in Subjects with Well-Controlled Type 2 Diabetes Mellitus. J Diabetes Res. 2015;2015:157698.
48. Chamarthi B, Ezrokhi M, Cincotta AH. Abstract 18968: Bromocriptine-QR: A Potential Novel Strategy for Cardiovascular Risk Reduction in Type 2 Diabetes. Circulation. 2013;128:A18968.
49. American Diabetes Association. 2008 Standards of Medical Care in Diabetes—2013. Diabetes Care. 2013;36:S12-54.
50. Nathan DM. Finding new treatments for diabetes—how many, how fast.... how good? N Engl J Med. 2007;356:437-40.
51. Food and Drug Administration (FDA). (2019). FDA approved drugs. [online] Available from http://www.centerwatch.co.uk/drug-information/fda-approvals/drug-details.aspx?DrugsID=1020. [Last accessed February, 2020].

FURTHER READINGS

1. Holt RIG, Barnett AH, Bailey CJ. Bromocriptine: old drug, new formulation and new indication. A review Diabetes Obes Metab. 2010;12:1048-57.
2. Chamarthi B and Cincotta AH. Effect of bromocriptine-QR therapy on glycemic control in subjects with type 2 diabetes mellitus whose dysglycemia is inadequately controlled on insulin. Postgrad med 2017;129:446-55.
3. Raskin P and Cincotta AH. Bromocriptine-QR therapy for the management of type 2 diabetes mellitus: developmental basis and therapeutic profile summary. Expert review endocrinology and metabolism 2016;11(2):113-48.

13

CHAPTER

Management of Dyslipidemia in Diabetes

Sailesh Lodha

INTRODUCTION

Diabetes has acquired epidemic proportions globally and in India. Current data indicate about 72 million population in India are affected with diabetes. Cardiovascular disease (CVD) is the leading cause of death in type 2 diabetes mellitus (T2DM) and about two-thirds of the people with diabetes aged 65 years or older succumb to CVD.[1,2] The risk of CVD increases two to four times in adults with diabetes.[2] Patients with diabetes have a two to four times increased risk for stroke and death from heart disease relative to patients without diabetes.[3] Diabetes is a CV risk equivalent. Dyslipidemia is a major contributing factor to atherosclerotic cardiovascular disease (ASCVD) and treating dyslipidemia improves CV outcomes.[4]

Thus, timely recognition and effective management of diabetic dyslipidemia (DD) to reach the desired goals and recommendations to set goal by various global and national associations are essential for preventing morbidity and mortality.

Dyslipidemia usually goes together with diabetes.[5] Diabetes and lipid metabolism are so interlinked that the term "diabetes lipidus" is suggested by some authors. ASCVD is associated with serum cholesterol and triglyceride (TG) levels in type 1 as well as in T2DM.[6,7] The risk of CVD is greater at any given level of serum cholesterol in patients with diabetes and its association with hypertriglyceridemia is stronger than in the general population.[8] There is compelling evidence in both, people with diabetes and people not affected with diabetes that reducing cholesterol significantly reduces CVD[9] and lower the better, there is no threshold below which a further reduction in low-density lipoprotein (LDL) cholesterol might be beneficial.[10]

Diabetes affected patients with a prior myocardial infarction (MI) are at a 2.5-fold greater risk of ASCVD events in future than in individuals with ASCVD without diabetes.[11] It has been argued since a long time whether patients with diabetes who have not had MIs should be treated as aggressively for cardiovascular risk factors as patients who have had MIs. Data from a Finnish population-based study suggested that individuals with T2DM and no history of MI have cardiovascular risk [fatal MI, nonfatal MI, cerebrovascular accident (CVA), or overall cardiovascular mortality] equivalent to those without diabetes and a history of MI.[12] In addition to hyperglycemia, individuals with T2DM have other risk factors like hypertension, low high-density lipoprotein cholesterol (HDL-C), high TG, small dense LDL cholesterol (LDL-C), a procoagulant state, and/or a proinflammatory milieu (**Table 13.1**). Based on this level of increased risk, the National Cholesterol Education Program Adult Treatment Panel III (NCEP ATP III) and the American Diabetes Association/American College of Cardiology (ADA/ACC) consensus statement considered individuals with T2DM to manifest an ASCVD equivalent (a 10-year risk of ASCVD events that is equal to that of individuals with established ASCVD) and therefore be at high risk.[13,14] According to the ADA and the ACC, people with diabetes with one or more additional risk factor should be considered as very high-risk category.[14]

Diabetic dyslipidemia is comprised of low HDL, high TG, and postprandial lipemia. In T2DM, LDL may not be elevated,[15] but the LDL is converted to smaller and more atherogenic lipoproteins—small dense LDL.[16] Hence, the LDL particle number is more. In the strong heart study, a 12% increase in CVD risk was observed in people with diabetes for every 10 mg/dL rise in LDL. This may also be seen in prediabetics also where insulin resistance is present with euglycemia. In a 7-year follow-up of San Antonio Heart Study, in which 195 of 1,734 subjects converted to T2DM, converters had significantly higher TG concentration and lower HDL-C than nonconverters.[17] This contributes to accelerated atherosclerosis in prediabetes. This view is supported by the action of some thiazolidinediones which lead to a greater improvement in lipid profiles than some other oral antidiabetic drugs (OADs).[18] DD results from effects of insulin on liver apoprotein production, regulation of lipoprotein lipase (LPL), actions of cholesteryl ester transfer protein (CETP), and other actions of insulin on adipose tissue and muscle, adipocytokines, and hyperglycemia.[19] Incretin activity also contributes to postprandial hypertriglyceridemia.

Low HDL-C is an independent factor for CVD, but it also contributes to the development of diabetes.[20] In type 1 diabetes mellitus (T1DM), hypertriglyceridemia may occur, but HDL-C levels are often normal or even high unless glycemic control is poor or nephropathy is present.[21] Qualitative abnormalities of lipoprotein kinetics are present in diabetes.[19] Increased TG synthesis by liver [occurring because of high circulating free fatty acids (FFAs)] is associated with increased secretion of apolipoprotein B (ApoB) (**Fig. 13.1**).[22]

TABLE 13.1: Key changes in lipoprotein metabolism in type 2 diabetes mellitus.

Lipoprotein	Quantitative changes	Qualitative changes	Kinetic/ metabolic changes
Chylomicron	• Increased plasma concentration	• Very few data (decreased ApoE content in rabbits with diabetes	• Increased production • Decreased catabolism
VLDL	• Increased plasma concentration	• Greater proportion of larger particles (VLDL1) • Increased palmitic acid-containing species and diacylglycerol, reduced sphingomyelin • Glycation	• Increased production • Decreased catabolism
LDL	• No change or slightly increased plasma concentration	• Greater proportion of small, dense particles (triacylglycerol enrichment) • Increased LDL oxidation • Increased palmitic acid-containing species and diacylglycerol, reduced sphingomyelin • Glycation	• Decreased catabolism
HDL	• Decreased plasma concentration	• Triacylglycerol enrichment • Reduced phospholipids, ApoE and ApoM • Glycation	• Increased catabolism

(ApoE: apolipoprotein E; HDL: high-density lipoprotein; LDL: low-density lipoprotein; VLDL: very low-density lipoprotein)

The intercellular transport of cholesterol and TG is mediated by lipoproteins. Insulin plays an important role in the metabolism of lipoproteins. ApoB is a component of chylomicrons, very low-density lipoprotein (VLDL), and LDL. Increased VLDL production is an important feature of insulin resistance.[23] There is decreased clearance of VLDL due to impaired activity of LPL.[19] Insulin is LPL inhibitor,[24] thus it

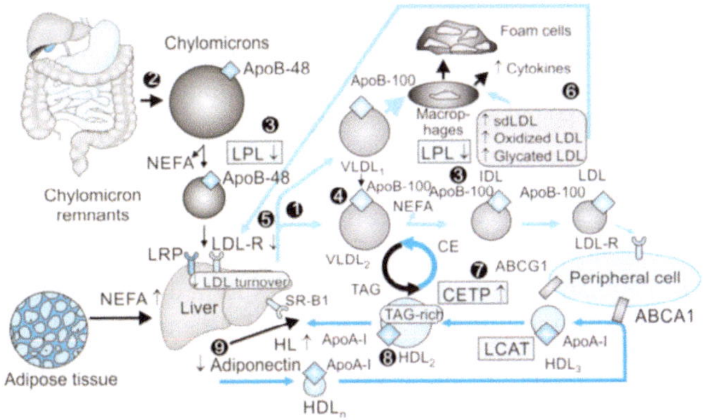

(CE: cholesterol ester; CETP: cholesteryl ester transfer protein; HDL: high-density lipoprotein; IDL: intermediate-density lipoprotein; LCAT: lecithin cholesterol acyltransferase; LDL: low-density lipoprotein; LPL: lipoprotein lipase; NEFA: nonesterified fatty acid; SR-B1: scavenger receptor B1; T2DM: type 2 diabetes mellitus; VLDL: very low-density lipoprotein)

FIG. 13.1: Main lipid abnormalities in T2DM. Triglycerides (hypertriglyceridemia, qualitative and kinetic abnormalities): (1) increased VLDL production (mostly VLDL1), (2) increased chylomicron production, (3) reduced catabolism of both chylomicrons and VLDLs (diminished LPL activity), and (4) increased production of large VLDL (VLDL1), preferentially taken up by macrophages; LDL (qualitative and kinetic abnormalities), (5) reduced LDL turnover (decreased LDL receptor), (6) increased number of glycated LDLs, small dense LDLs (triglycerides rich), and oxidized LDLs, which are preferentially taken up by macrophages; HDL (low HDLcholesterol, qualitative and kinetic abnormalities), (7) increased CETP activity (increased transfer of triglycerides from lipoproteins to LDLs and HDLs), (8) increased triglycerides content of HDLs, promoting HL activity and HDL catabolism, and (9) low plasma adiponectin favoring the increase in HDL catabolism.

Source: Modified from Vergès B. Pathophysiology of diabetic dyslipidaemia: where are we? Diabetologia. 2015;58(5):886-99.

regulates the amount of circulating FFAs. In the fed state, high levels of insulin promote TG uptake by adipocytes where they are stored. But in fasting when insulin concentration is low, FFAs are released by adipocytes and transported to liver. In hepatocytes under the influence of insulin, production of TG and glycogen is stimulated. Insulin inhibits the transcription of microsomal TG transfer protein, which mediates the transfer of TGs to nascent ApoB.

Insulin also inhibits glucose production and secretion of ApoB. Insulin regulates ApoB via multiple complex mechanisms. T2DM is associated with overproduction of ApoB and its reduced clearance. Glycated ApoB is double even in well-controlled diabetes.[25] Postprandial lipemia results from lowered LPL activity. In the presence of other features of metabolic syndrome, hypertriglyceridemia promotes the development of T2DM. It also predicts CHD risk, independently of other risk factors.[6] An increase of TG-rich lipoproteins is associated with low HDL and high small dense LDL. There is transfer of TG in the opposite direction such that cholesteryl ester-depleted HDL and LDL becomes TG-rich. Glycated LDL is more susceptible to oxidation. Glycation of LDL decreases its LDL receptor-mediated catabolism. The antioxidative and anti-inflammatory effects of HDL are reduced in diabetes.[26] Glycation of HDL enhances its catabolism.

CLINICAL INVESTIGATIONS

Triad of low HDL, high TGs, and postprandial lipemia form DD. The relatively normal cholesterol levels in diabetes hide an atherogenic lipid profile.[27] This is more characteristically seen in the "Asian Indian phenotype" or thin fat Indian with higher visceral fat, higher small dense LDL, and low HDL with high TG. Postprandial lipemia is characterized by a rise in TG-rich lipoproteins with food consumption.

Low-density lipoprotein cholesterol in many patients with diabetes is within normal limits, but the particle size is smaller and dense (higher ApoB) and the clearance of these small dense particles is slower.[28] Hence, estimating ApoB measurement is a better discriminating index of therapeutic response or atherogenic risk than LDL-C. In the DCCT (Diabetes Control and Complications Trial), intensive treatment of diabetes had no significant effect on LDL and HDL-C levels, rather there was a decreased ApoB and lipoprotein(a) and with favorable alterations in lipoprotein subclasses. These alterations may not be apparent by standard lipid profile. Obviously, these changes will have implications for the progression of microvascular and macrovascular complications. The LDL-C in diabetes also underestimates the atherogenic contribution of TG-rich particles. Thus, non-HDL-C is a better measure of atherogenicity in diabetes.[29] As ApoB measurement is very expensive at present and may not be widely available, non-HDL-C estimation can serve the purpose to a large extent. There is consensus on LDL <100 mg/dL (2.6 mmol/L) for patients with diabetes without additional cardiovascular risk. For patients with diabetes who are at a higher risk with additional cardiovascular risk factors, a target of LDL <70 mg/dL (1.8 mmol/L) should be aimed. If this cannot be achieved, lowering LDL 30–40% (ADA) or ≥50% [European Society of Cardiology/European Association for the Study of Diabetes (ESC/EASD)] from baseline is targeted.

Non-HDL-C and ApoB are considered as secondary treatment goals because there is insufficient evidence to show that lowering non-HDL-C and ApoB is superior to LDL lowering in terms of improving cardiovascular outcomes. The ADA recommends a treatment target of non-HDL-C <100 mg/dL (2.6 mmol/L) and <130 mg/dL (3.4 mmol/L) for patients with diabetes with and without an additional CVD risk factor, respectively. Targets for ApoB are <80 mg/dL and <90 mg/dL for those with and without an additional CVD risk factor, respectively. Similarly, TG and HDL-C are also secondary treatment targets. The recommended treatment goals are TGs <150 mg/dL

(1.7 mmol/L) and HDL >40 mg/dL (1.0 mmol/L) in men and >50 mg/dL (1.3 mmol/L) in women.[30] Periodic monitoring for compliance and efficacy of the treatment is required however the need and timing should be based on clinical judgment.

In the current scenario, CV risk reduction in patients with diabetes can be done by lifestyle alterations (physical activity, proper nutrition, cessation of alcohol and tobacco), controlling hyperglycemia, hypertension, and dyslipidemia. In obese or overweight individuals, weight loss is very helpful. Moderate weight loss (5% of body weight) has shown many benefits ranging from increasing insulin sensitivity, improving glycemic control, and lipid parameters.[31] A recent primary care-based trial in the UK [DiRECT (Diabetes Remission Clinical Trial)][32] has shown complete reversal of diabetes in half of the participants by weight reduction in early course of T2DM.

MEDICAL NUTRITION THERAPY

Medical nutrition therapy for DD comprises a diet plan which takes into consideration patients liking and disliking along with the lipid and glycemic targets. Adequate fiber intake and a low-fat diet improved lipid profiles, with fiber reducing inflammatory markers[33] and the low-fat diet lowering HDL-C levels. Omega-3 fatty acids significantly increased HDL-C and reduced VLDL-TG.[34]

What should be the percentage of carbohydrates, fats, and proteins in the menu of people with diabetes is controversial. Recently, more weightage is given to carbohydrate restriction and now their contribution to the calories below 60–65% is widely accepted. Guidance on sources of the nutrients should be emphasized: Raw vegetables, fresh fruits, dairy products, whole grain, and legumes should form the source of carbohydrates. Sources that contain added fat, sugar, and sodium should be avoided; leaner protein sources and meat alternatives are preferred; vegetarians can derive proteins from nuts, pulses, and beans. Dietary fat should be mainly composed of monounsaturated and polyunsaturated fats instead of saturated and trans fat. For individuals who consume alcohol, moderate consumption (≤ one drink/day for women and ≤ two drinks/day for men) has been advised.[35] There is robust evidence that low levels of alcohol intake do not provide any protective health benefits. Any level of alcohol consumption can be associated with range of cancers and there is no justification for drinking for health reasons. Alcohol is a common cause of hypertriglyceridemia.

Consumption of nuts and seeds is also beneficial for reducing TGs, LDL, and increasing HDL. Different dietary patterns in the management of T2DM have concluded that low-carbohydrate, low-glycemic index diet consumption, and Mediterranean and high-protein consumption showed better glycemic control. Maximum benefits were with Mediterranean diet. It is desirable to increase HDL to 45 or greater. Although this may be an ideal goal for many patients and their physicians, it is impractical. At present, there is no effective drug for increasing HDL. The only effective measures are stopping smoking and increasing physical activity with or without weight loss. Ironically, diets low in cholesterol and saturated fats tend to decrease HDL. Effect of exercise on the components of DD is favorable. Compared with the control trial, exercise reduced postprandial lipemia by a mean of 20% ($p < 0.05$), whereas intake restriction reduced it by 7% (NS). This study highlighted that the effect of exercise on postprandial lipids was much more and different from that attributable to the energy deficit incurred.[36]

Glycemic control itself with or without insulin can improve dyslipidemia to a great extent. Metformin decreases serum TGs and improves insulin resistance. Other drugs used in the management of diabetes may also have minor effects on lipid metabolism. Pioglitazone can increase the particle size of LDL and a small favorable effect on TG and HDL. The small but statistically insignificant increase in LDL cholesterol may occur following treatment with sodium-glucose cotransporter-2 (SGLT-2) inhibitors but the ratio of LDL to HDL is unaltered. This suggests that the dramatic improvement in CV outcomes with empagliflozin is unrelated to the effects on dyslipidemia.[37]

STATINS

Statin is the first agent for dyslipidemia in patients with diabetes and people not with diabetes. Although their main effect is on LDL reduction, they also have a modest effect on lowering TG and raising HDL.

Statins inhibit the rate-limiting enzyme in cholesterol biosynthesis which is 3-hydroxy-3-methylglutaryl coenzyme A (HMG-CoA). There is enormous data which clearly show that lowering cholesterol can reduce CV mortality. They are strongly recommended by all the current guidelines for CV risk reduction.[38] Based on various guidelines, moderate-intensity statins are recommended in all patients with diabetes aged 40–75 years with LDL-C values between 70 and 189 mg/dL and high-intensity statins in those with previous events or acute coronary syndrome (ACS) or a ≥7.5% estimated 10-year risk for ASCVD.

Epidemiologic studies show exceedingly increased susceptibility for ASCVD in patients with T2DM. Similar susceptibility level is seen in T1DM patients in whom the disease prolongs beyond a period of 15 years or those who show two or more major CV risk factors. Three placebo-controlled, primary prevention trials were conducted in T2DM patients with moderate-intensity statin dosage. Either atorvastatin

10 mg/day or simvastatin 40 mg/day was administered on a daily basis.

- The *CARDS (Collaborative Atorvastatin Diabetes Study)*: Primary prevention of CVD with atorvastatin in T2DM.
- The ASCOT–LLA (Anglo-Scandinavian Cardiac Outcomes Trial–Lipid-lowering Arm).
- The Heart Protection Study (HPS) of cholesterol lowering with simvastatin.

All the trials showed considerable decrease in cardiovascular complication in the subjects, thereby showing strong evidence in favor of statin administration in T2DM patients as a lipid-lowering agent. In diabetes therapy, the predominance of statins is similar to the same effect with metformin.

Another concept which is similar but expressed in other words is the "rule of 6" phenomenon,[39] which mentions an extra 6% decrease in LDL-C with the statin dosage being doubled every time. Though rhabdomyolysis is very infrequent, an additional decrease is significant as increased dosage of statin may enhance chances of myalgias, thereby causing to stop the drug totally. Over 14 random trials[5] were conducted in a total of 18,686 people with diabetes. The meta-analysis, which comprised of 1,466 T1DM patients and 17,220 T2DM patients, presented 9% decrease in mortality in all possibilities for every 1 mmol/L decrease in LDL-C.

The foremost substantial primary prevention study to observe the statin effect particularly on the basis of cardiovascular comorbidities is the CARDS. The study was conducted in T2DM patients in the absence of preexisting CVD (n = 2838) by administering 10 mg atorvastatin everyday.[9] The outcome estimated a 40%, 37%, and 48% lowering of LDL-C levels, reduced major CV complications, and decreased occurrence of stroke, respectively. The most extensive trial regarding statin usage is the HPS. The study comprised diabetes (N ¼ 5,963, 90% T2DM) who were administered 40 mg simvastatin on a daily basis had an outcome of 33% reduction in LDL-C levels and 31% decrease in CV complications. The recommended therapy for DD is the administration of statins as per guidelines. Situation of optimal statin use in developing and underdeveloped countries may be the same or perhaps worse. In one of the largest statin prescription studies, statins were prescribed in only half of the clinic-based patients in India with T2DM. Prescription of high-dose statins was shown to be very low.[40] Taiwanese nationwide diabetes database have shown that statin therapy was associated with a 25% lower rate of lower-extremity amputations and a 22% risk reduction of CV mortality.

Undoubtedly, statins substantially reduce CV events, but still 60–75% of patients on statins have CV events as it has been shown in a large number of clinical trials.[41] This could be due to intervention that is too late, too brief, or due to inadequate

LDL-C lowering. Even with effective statin therapy, residual risk remains which, to some extent, can be tackled by nonstatin lipid-lowering drugs like fibrates which are known to have an effect on increasing LDL particle size.

Statin-induced Diabetes Mellitus and Muscle Toxicity

The Food and Drug Administration (FDA) sounded an alarm in 2012 for a noticeable increase in glycated hemoglobin (HbA1c) and fasting glucose with statin use. Preiss et al.[42] in a meta-analysis estimated that in patients with prior CV event, intensive statin therapy will prevent around three new events per year in ~500 subjects and at the same time with one additional case of diabetes. Ridker et al. reported in the JUPITER (Justification for the Use of Statins in Primary Prevention: an Intervention Trial Evaluating Rosuvastatin) trial[43] which included 17,802 subjects that despite a 26% increase in the relative risk for new diabetes with rosuvastatin 20 mg, the major CVD event rate reduction was 44% in those who developed diabetes. Data on pravastatin, however, are conflicting. The risk of new diabetes is dose dependent, greater in elderly individuals, and is a class effect. The proposed mechanisms are—decreased expression of glucose transporter type 2 (GLUT2), increased insulin resistance (decreased GLUT4 expression in adipocytes), decreased insulin sensitivity, decreased adiponectin, and mitochondrial dysfunction by reduced coenzyme Q-mediated adenosine triphosphate (ATP) production. Statin-induced myalgias and myopathy can aggravate sarcopenia which can hamper physical activity.

In the light of a minor increase in new-onset diabetes, statin treatment, however, should not be withheld wherever it is indicated, especially in those at high risk of CVD. In addition to their potent lipid-lowering efficacy, statins have many pleiotropic benefits like stabilization of coronary plaques, improvement in proteinuria, reduction of retinal exudates, increase in bone mineral density, antioxidant/anti-inflammatory effects, and possibly a reduced incidence of dementia. Unlike atorvastatin, other statins require minor dose adjustments in renal failure.

Apart from lifestyle alterations, guidelines recommend attaining normal glycemic control with high-intensity statin therapy. The high-intensity statin dosages like atorvastatin 40–80 mg or rosuvastatin 20–40 mg are prescribed across all age groups in those apparent CHD. The same therapy is also recommended in patients between 40 and 75 years of age with increased risk factors. A moderate-intensity statin therapy with atorvastatin 10–20 mg or simvastatin 20–40 mg is recommended in those above 40 years of age in the absence of other risk factors. Clinical judgment should guide the use of moderate- or high-intensity statin therapy in patients younger than 40 years or older than 75 years with additional risk factors. For patients <40 years and >75 years with other risk factors, clinical judgment should be utilized to use statins.

Statin-induced Myotoxicity

It is one of the severe adverse effects of statins. It can manifest in mild form as myalgias or may progress to myositis and the most severe form like rhabdomyolysis. Mild elevations of liver transaminases are common without any hepatic damage. Patients with underlying liver or renal disease and elderly patients or who are on multiple medications may have more severe reactions. An increase in creatine phosphokinase (CPK) which is released from skeletal muscle is noted in about 10% of patients.[44] HMG-CoA reductase inhibitors are metabolized by the cytochrome P450 system; drugs that inhibit cytochrome P450 activity increase the risk of hepatotoxicity and myopathy. There are studies which prove the teratogenicity of HMG-CoA reductase inhibitors. Hence, they are not prescribed in pregnant women.

Generally, these symptoms occur after 4 weeks of starting or intensification of treatment. About 1.5–5% of patients present with muscle-related symptoms. The PRIMO (Prediction of Muscular Risk in Observational Conditions) study claimed that the statin-induced muscle symptoms are underestimated. Patients should be counseled for reporting muscle discomfort or muscle aches. CPK measurement is not required in asymptomatic patients. This is needed only when symptoms are present. Statin-induced myopathy could present as only myalgia with mild elevations of CPK or myositis with CPK elevations >10 times of upper limit of normal (ULN). Very rarely, it can present as rhabdomyolysis which is associated with CPK >10,000 IU/L and rise in serum creatinine. If CPK levels are <10 times the ULN, then statin therapy may be continued in same or reduced doses with a watch on symptoms. If CPK levels >10,000 IU/L or above 10 times the ULN, then patient should be admitted for intravenous hydration to avoid renal damage by preventing rhabdomyolysis. If muscle symptoms are intense, statin should be withdrawn or may be given in a reduced dose or replaced by a different agent whenever clinically feasible. In patients with no symptoms, if liver enzymes are between one and three times the ULN, statin may be continued. If levels increase > three times the ULN, then reduce the statin dose or discontinue treatment and also search for other possible etiologies. The mechanism of this myopathy is not clear, but few theories proposed are—reduced levels of coenzyme Q10 leading to mitochondrial dysfunction, isoprenoids are also depleted which are another product of the same mevalonate pathway and this may promote muscle apoptosis, and muscle membrane cholesterol may be lowered.

Patients who are prone for statin-induced muscle toxicity are elderly, those on concomitant therapy with fibrates, erythromycin, or azole antifungals. Vitamin D deficiency is a common cause. Other reasons could be small body habitus, a family history of statin myotoxicity, renal impairment, infection, trauma, alcohol abuse, and untreated hypothyroidism.

Proprotein Convertase Subtilisin/Kexin Type 9 Inhibitors

Cholesterol metabolism can be balanced crucially by sterol regulatory element-binding protein 2 (SREBP-2). Low-density lipoprotein receptor (LDLR) degradation can be controlled by proprotein convertase subtilisin/kexin type 9 (PCSK9). PCSK9, a hepatic protease, combines to and internalizes LDLR into lysosomes thereby aiding their destruction. The monoclonal antibodies that can inactivate this PCSK9 are evolocumab and alirocumab. By stopping LDLR destroying, LDL-C levels may be reduced up to 50–60% more than the level attained by only statin therapy. PCSK9 inhibitors are the newly developed group of exciting agents which are recommended for decreasing LDL-C marking the latest phase in lipid-lowering therapy. Some adverse effects could be nasopharyngitis (11.3% vs. 11.1% in placebo), itching and erythema-like effects at injection site, swelling, pain or tenderness, and influenza, urinary tract infection, diarrhea, bronchitis, myalgia, muscle spasms, sinusitis, cough, and musculoskeletal pain.

EZETIMIBE

Ezetimibe acts locally in small intestine by blocking the absorption of dietary cholesterol as well as prevention of the reabsorption of cholesterol entering the small intestine with bile. It reduces the cholesterol supply to liver cells which then derive it from circulation thereby decreasing the circulatory cholesterol. Ezetimibe is concentrated in the jejunal enterocytes brush border, where it inhibits cholesterol absorption by a process which involves binding to cholesterol transport protein—Niemann-Pick C1-Like 1 protein.[45] The IMPROVE-IT (Improved Reduction of Outcomes: Vytorin Efficacy International Trial) has shown the safety and efficacy of ezetimibe which was considered as controversial earlier. When statin alone is not sufficient or in statin intolerance, it serves as an adjuvant therapy or a monotherapy and provides incremental LDL lowering in diabetes. It is safe and well-tolerated. It may increase liver enzymes too like statins but when used in combination with statins, it does not significantly cause an increase in liver enzymes more than is observed with statin therapy alone.

BILE ACID SEQUESTRANTS

In patients who cannot tolerate statins, a bile acid sequestrant (BAS) can be utilized for LDL lowering. BAS like colesevelam is suitable for pregnancy and children where statins are contraindicated. Colesevelam can lower LDL-C, but it can increase TG by about 15% and has lesser gastrointestinal side effects than other drugs from this family. It can also serve as a weak antihyperglycemic agent by reducing HbA1c by 0.5%.[46] BAS is contraindicated in moderate-to-severe hypertriglyceridemia and dysbetalipoproteinemia.

SAROGLITAZAR

Drugs with agonistic activity on both peroxisome proliferator-activated receptor-α (PPAR-α) and PPAR-γ are being researched since last many decades. Possibility of controlling glucose and lipid parameters by a single agent is actively pursued. This class of antidiabetic-/lipid-lowering drug is called "glitazar". Out of so many dual PPAR-α and PPAR-γ agonists which were clinically developed, none could progress beyond phase III development due to poor efficacy or safety issues. Saroglitazar is one such molecule which appears to have passed these hurdles. It has a strong PPAR-α with moderate PPAR-γ action. Saroglitazar is the first glitazar to receive marketing approval in India recently. Large international data is not available yet. At present, it is available as 4 mg tablet. It is a dual PPAR-α and PPAR-γ agonist with a predominant alpha agonistic activity through which it reduces TGs and also has a modest glucose-lowering activity through its gamma agonistic activity.[47] It has no adverse effects related to kidney and muscle. Gastritis, dyspepsia, asthenia, and pyrexia are the most common side effects. It can be used as an adjunct to statins and fibrates for controlling hypertriglyceridemia. It can also be used as an adjunct in rare situations where TG lowering is not possible with all the currently available agents.[48]

Fibrates act through PPAR-α receptor agonistic activity to reduce TG. They have a small effect on LDL lowering. Statin is the established treatment regimen for a person with diabetes, however, it alone is insufficient many times to normalize persistently high TG. Fibrates are best suited for this situation as an add-on to statin. How much benefit is obtained by lowering TG is not clear. In the MIRACL (Myocardial Ischemia Reduction with Aggressive Cholesterol Lowering) and dal-OUTCOMES studies, fasting TG predicted recurrent ischemic events in patients with ACS treated with statins and it indicated a strong association of fasting TG with residual risk after ACS in patients receiving adequate statin. The BIP (Bezafibrate Infarction Prevention) trial failed to show a reduction in primary cardiovascular endpoints. A 16–29% risk reduction in vascular events has been demonstrated in a meta-analysis of six major randomized controlled trials[49] dealing with fibrates in various lipid disorders, but CV events did not decline consistently. The potential of combining fibrate with statin for therapy of residual CVR in people with diabetes who are only on simvastatin was studied by the ACCORD (Action to Control Cardiovascular Risk in Diabetes)-lipid trial. The outcome presented a considerable 28.5% (from 17.32 to 12.37) lowering in cardiovascular comorbidities only in a part of patients who are in the highest tertile with TG (>2.3 mmol/L) and HDL-C in the lowest tertile (0.88 mmol/L).

The ADA does not support fibrate only therapy for CVR reduction in T2DM patients. The ADA favors statin plus fibrate in men with both TG >204 mg/dL (2.3 mmol/L) and HDL-C <34 mg/dL (0.9 mmol/L). The American Heart Association (AHA) is more conservative as it approves fibrate only when TG levels are >500 mg/dL (>5.65 mmol/L).

The VA-HIT (Veterans Affairs High-density Lipoprotein Cholesterol Intervention Trial) showed that gemfibrozil therapy can reduce the risk of major CV events in patients with primary lipid abnormality of low HDL. It suggested that by reducing TG and raising HDL, CV events can be reduced.[50] A target HDL of 45 mg/dL though may be ideal but it is generally impractical as such a goal is usually nonachievable and the benefits of such a goal are unproven. Fibrates can be used to treat isolated hypertriglyceridemia. Chances of acute pancreatitis rise markedly after TG of >1,000 mg/dL, hence lowering TG prevents this dreaded complication. Combining fibrates with statin can be contemplated depending on each patient. The patients who are susceptible to increased TG levels and reduced HDL improve with the recommendation of combination therapy. But administering fibrate along with statin comes with more chances of myopathy and rhabdomyolysis, particularly when gemfibrozil is taken with statin; hence, utmost care should be exercised while prescribing them together. The tolerability is favorable when statin is given along with fenofibrate or bezafibrate than when combined with gemfibrozil. Such combinations, however, are avoided in diabetes related kidney disease.

NIACIN

Niacin is an independent efficient drug to increase HDL levels.[51] When the patient responds well to the drug, one can expect a 25% increase in HDL levels, though it may not be sufficient to increase lower HDL levels to attain the required target level. Niacin is being rarely prescribed in patients with diabetes , but mostly averted as it may aggravate hyperglycemia. Though fibric acids and statins enhance HDL levels, it is only to a moderate extent when compared to the levels increased by niacin. The VA-HIT trial and subgroup analyses of fibric acid confirm that therapy for increased TGs is advantageous. Apart from niacin, fibric acids, statins at very heavy doses, and fish oil seem to decrease TG levels. Combining statins and niacin for therapy of T2DM patients can possibly be restricted for high-risk hypertriglyceridemia-related pancreatitis subjects as there is not many studies and information present till now.

BARIATRIC SURGERY

Bariatric procedure or "metabolic surgery" is the treatment of choice as per the guidelines of the International Diabetes Federation Taskforce for obese patient who have uncontrolled diabetes and a body mass index (BMI) >30 kg/m^2. The surgery is also indicated by the ADA and the AHA/ACC/Obesity Society if patient's BMI >35 kg/m^2. A meta-analysis done for a mean follow-up of 57.8 months period presented an outcome of 65% of exemption from hyperlipidemia.[52] The STAMPEDE (Systemic Therapy in Advancing or Metastatic Prostate Cancer: Evaluation of Drug Efficacy) trial with a 3-year follow-up in[53] patients who elected the bariatric Roux-en-Y gastric bypass or sleeve gastrectomy showed a considerably higher reduction in TG levels (mean 41.9% and 31.5%, respectively) and greatly enhanced HDL-C levels (mean 34.7% and 35%, respectively) when compared to subjects who are administered only medicines; nevertheless, a very little amount of LDL-C level increase was observed. A follow-up was done in patients with diabetes where a general reduction in cardiovascular mortality for over a period of 10 years was observed in the Swedish Obese Subjects study.

Patients with diabetes generally show typically less HDL levels and increased TG levels with "optimal" LDL levels, yet the crucial point in treatment continues to be decreasing LDL levels. Most of the patients with diabetes show generalized lipid particle abnormalities. The patient presents with increased LDL level simultaneously with decreased HDL and more TG levels. Decreasing the LDL level is the most crucial part of treatment. Once the LDL target level is attained, the treatment should proceed further with optimizing the HDL and TG levels. This approach is not followed in patients with dangerously increased TG levels (>500 mg/dL) who are prone to pancreatitis. In such cases, treatment is first targeted toward increased TGs to make it normal.

More lipid modulating drugs have to be evolved. Also, more new molecules have to be developed to avoid adverse effects of statins like myopathy and mild glucose increase. The frequently strived molecules are the CETP and the PCSK9 inhibitors. More recently explored molecules such as ApoB synthesis inhibitors and microsomal triglyceride transfer protein (MTTP) inhibitors are studied in patients with familial hypercholesterolemia for being used in patients with diabetes as they may interest the researchers to study them as time comes.

CONCLUSION

Patients with diabetes carry a high CV risk even with a normal LDL. Although high TG and low HDL are the peculiarities of DD, LDL lowering remains a priority. Lowering TG or raising HDL may not be so beneficial and this is surrounded by controversies. Hence, first priority is LDL lowering which can be followed by measures to lower TG and raising HDL. Lifestyle measures alone usually fail. Statins form the mainstay of treatment of DD. All guidelines recommend aggressive statin use in people with diabetes . At present, statins are safe and effective in preventing CVD in patients with diabetes. In future, more effective and safer agents will be available.

REFERENCES

1. Jaiswal M, Schinske A, Pop-Busui R. Lipids and lipid management in diabetes. Best Pract Res Clin Endocrinol Metab. 2014;28(3):325-38.
2. Cardiovacular Disease and Diabetes. American Heart Association Website. http://www.heart.org/HEARTORG/Conditions/Diabetes/WhyDia betesMatters/Cardiovascular-Disease-Diabetes_UCM_313865_Article. jsp/.VqfJL5orKUk. Accessed 2601.16.
3. Wu L, Parhofer KG. Diabetic dyslipidemia. Metabolism. 2014;63(12):1469-79.
4. Cholesterol Treatment Trialists' (CTT) Collaboration, Baigent C, Blackwell L, et al. Efficacy and safety of more intensive lowering of LDL cholesterol: a meta-analysis of data from 170,000 participants in 26 randomised trials. Lancet. 2010;376(9753):1670-81.
5. Chapman MJ, Ginsberg HN, Amarenco P, et al. Triglyceride-rich lipoproteins and high-density lipoprotein cholesterol in patients at high risk of cardiovascular disease: evidence and guidance for management. Eur Heart J. 2011;32:1345-61.
6. West KM, Ahuja MM, Bennett PH, et al. The role of circulating glucose and triglyceride concentrations and their interactions with other "risk factors" as determinants of arterial disease in nine diabetic population samples from the WHO multinational study. Diabetes Care. 1983;6:361-9.
7. Howard BV, Robbins DC, Sievers ML, et al. LDL cholesterol as a strong predictor of coronary heart disease in diabetic individuals with insulin resistance and low LDL: the Strong Heart Study. Arterioscler Thromb Vasc Biol. 2000;20:830-5.
8. Stamler J, Vaccaro O, Neaton JD, Wentworth D. Diabetes, other risk factors, and 12-yr cardiovascular mortality for men screened in the Multiple Risk Factor Intervention Trial. Diabetes Care. 1993;16:434-44.
9. Colhoun HM, Betteridge DJ, Durrington PN, et al. Primary prevention of cardiovascular disease with atorvastatin in type 2 diabetes in the collaborative atorvastatin diabetes study (CARDS): multicentre randomised placebo-controlled trial. Lancet. 2004;364:685-96.
10. Baigent C, Keech A, Kearney PM, et al. Efficacy and safety of cholesterol-lowering treatment: prospective meta-analysis of data from 90,056 participants in 14 randomised trials of statins. Lancet. 2005;366:1267-78.

11. Haffner SM. Management of dyslipidemia in adults with diabetes. Diabetes Care. 1998;21:160-78.
12. Haffner SM, Lehto S, Rönnemaa T, Pyörälä K, Laakso M. Mortality from coronary heart disease in subjects with type 2 diabetes and in nondiabetic subjects with and without prior myocardial infarction. N Engl J Med. 1998;339:229-34.
13. National Institutes of Health; National Heart Lung, and Blood Institute; 2002 National Cholesterol Education Program. Third report of the National Cholesterol Education Program (NCEP) Expert Panel on detection, evaluation, and treatment of high blood cholesterol in adults (Adult Treatment Panel III): Final Report. NIH Publication No. 02-5215. September 2002.
14. Brunzell JD, Davidson M, Furberg CD, et al. Lipoprotein management in patients with cardiometabolic risk: consensus statement from the American Diabetes Association and the American College of Cardiology Foundation. Diabetes Care. 2008;31:811-22.
15. Cowie CC, Howard BV, Harris MI. Serum lipoproteins in African Americans and Whites with non-insulin-dependent diabetes in the US population. Circulation. 1994;90:1185-93.
16. Krauss RM. Heterogeneity of plasma low-density lipoproteins and atherosclerosis risk. Curr Opin Lipidol. 1994;5:339-49.
17. Haffner SM, Mykkanen L, Festa A, Burke JP, Stern MP. Insulin-resistant prediabetic subjects have more atherogenic risk factors than insulin-sensitive prediabetic subjects: implications for preventing coronary heart disease during the prediabetic state. Circulation. 2000;101:975-80.
18. Ginsberg H, Plutzky J, Sobel BE. A review of metabolic and cardiovascular effects of oral antidiabetic agents: beyond glucose-level lowering. J Cardiovasc Risk. 1999;6:337-46.
19. Taskinen MR. Diabetic dyslipidaemia: from basic research to clinical practice. Diabetologia. 2003;46:733-49.
20. Abbasi A, Corpeleijn E, Gansevoort RT, et al. Role of HDL cholesterol and estimates of HDL particle composition in future development of type 2 diabetes in the general population: the PREVEND study. J Clin Endocrinol Metab. 2013;98:E1352-9.
21. Dean JD, Durrington PN. Treatment of dyslipoproteinaemia in diabetes mellitus. Diabet Med. 1996.
22. Warraich HJ, Wong ND, Rana JS. Role for combination therapy in diabetic dyslipidemia. Curr Cardiol Rep. 2015;17:32.
23. McEneny J, O'Kane MJ, Moles KW, et al. Very low density lipoprotein subfractions in type II diabetes mellitus: alterations in composition and susceptibility to oxidation. Diabetologia. 2000;43:485-93.
24. Nikkila EA, Kekki M. Plasma triglyceride transport kinetics in diabetes mellitus. Metabolism. 1973;22:1-22.
25. Tames FJ, Mackness MI, Arrol S, Laing I, Durrington PN. Non-enzymatic glycation of apolipoprotein B in the sera of diabetic and non-diabetic subjects. Atherosclerosis. 1992;93:237-44.
26. Morgantini C, Natali A, Boldrini B, et al. Anti-inflammatory and antioxidant properties of HDLs are impaired in type 2 diabetes. Diabetes. 2011;60:2617-23.
27. Jenkins AJ, Best JD, Klein RL, Lyons TJ. Lipoproteins, glycoxidation and diabetic angiopathy. Diabetes Metab Res Rev. 2004;20:349-68.
28. Chapman MJ, Ginsberg HN, Amarenco P, et al. Triglyceride-rich lipoproteins and high-density lipoprotein cholesterol in patients at high risk of cardiovascular disease: evidence and guidance for management. Eur Heart J. 2011;32:1345-61.
29. Emerging Risk Factors Collaboration, Di Angelantonio E, Sarwar N, et al. Major lipids, apolipoproteins, and risk of vascular disease. JAMA. 2009;302:1993-2000.

30. American Diabetes A. Standards of medical care in diabetes—2013. Diabetes Care 2013;36(Suppl 1):S11-66.
31. Klein S, Sheard NF, Pi-Sunyer X, et al. Weight management through lifestyle modification for the prevention and management of type 2 diabetes: rationale and strategies. A statement of the American Diabetes Association, the North American Association for the Study of Obesity, and the American Society for Clinical Nutrition. Am J Clin Nutr. 2004;80(2):257-63.
32. Primary care-led weight management for remission of type 2 diabetes (DiRECT): an open-label, cluster-randomised trial . Michael EJ Lean, Wilma S Leslie, Alison C Barnes et al. lancet 2018, 391,10120, 541-51 .
33. Wheeler ML, Dunbar SA, Jaacks LM, et al. Macronutrients, food groups, and eating patterns in the management of diabetes: a systematic review of the literature, 2010. Diabetes Care 2012;35:434e45.
34. Bosch J, Gerstein HC, Dagenais GR, et al. n-3 fatty acids and cardiovascular outcomes in patients with dysglycaemia. N Engl J Med 2012;367:309e18.
35. Evert AB, Boucher JL, Cypress M, et al. Nutrition therapy recommendations for the management of adults with diabetes. Diabetes Care. 2013;36(11): 3821-42.
36. Gill JM, Hardman AE. Postprandial lipemia: effects of exercise and restriction of energy intake compared. Am J Clin Nutr. 2000;71(2):465-71.
37. Zinman B, Wanner C, Lachin JM, et al. Empagliflozin, cardiovascular outcomes, and mortality in type 2 diabetes. N Engl J Med. 2015;373:2117-28.
38. American Diabetes Association. Standards of medical care in diabetes. Diabetes Care. 2016;1(Suppl 1):S62-S3.
39. Bays H, Stein EA. Pharmacotherapy for dyslipidaemia—current therapies and future agents. Expert Opin Pharmacother. 2003;4(11):1901-38.
40. Gupta R, Lodha S, Sharma KK, et al. Evaluation of statin prescriptions in type 2 diabetes: India Heart Watch-2. BMJ Open Diabetes Research and Care 2016;4: e000275. doi:10.1136/bmjdrc-2016-000275.
41. Libby P. The forgotten majority: unfinished business in cardiovascular risk reduction. J Am Coll Cardiol. 2005;46(7):1225-8.
42. Risk of incident diabetes with intensive-dose compared with moderate-dose statin therapy: a meta-analysis.D Preiss, SRK Seshasai, P Welsh, JAMA 2011 Jun 22;305(24):2556-64.
43. Ridker PM, Pradhan A, MacFadyen JG, et al. Cardiovascular benefits and diabetes risks of statin therapy in primary prevention: an analysis from the JUPITER trial. Lancet. 2012;380(9841):565-71.
44. Tomaszewski M, Stępień KM, Tomaszewska J, Czuczwar SJ. Statin-induced myopathies. Pharmacol Rep. 2011;63(4):859-66.
45. Garcia-Calvo M, Lisnock J, Bull HG, et al. The target of ezetimibe is Niemann-Pick C1-Like 1 (NPC1L1). Proc Natl Acad Sci USA. 2005;102:8132-7.
46. Younk LM, Davis SN. Evaluation of colesevelam hydrochloride for the treatment of type 2 diabetes. Expert Opin Drug Metab Toxicol 2012;8:515e25.
47. Jani, R. H. et al. A multicenter, prospective, randomized, double-blind study to evaluate the safety and efficacy of Saroglitazar 2 and 4 mg compared with placebo in type 2 diabetes mellitus patients having hypertriglyceridemia not controlled with atorvastatin therapy (PRESS VI). Diabetes Technol Ther. 2014;16:63-71.
48. Lodha S, et al. Severe hypertriglyceridaemia in an adolescent with lipoprotein lipase deficiency: responding to triple drug combination., ePoster # 657, EASD Munich, 2016.
49. Lee M, Saver JL, Towfighi A, et al. Efficacy of fibrates for cardiovascular risk reduction in persons with atherogenic dyslipidaemia: a meta-analysis. Atherosclerosis 2011;217:492e8.
50. Rubins HB, Robins SJ, Collins D, et al. Gemfibrozil for the secondary prevention of coronary heart disease in men with low levels of high-density lipoprotein cholesterol. Veterans Affairs High-Density Lipoprotein Cholesterol Intervention Trial Study Group. N Engl J Med. 1999;341(6):410-8.

51. Rader DJ. Pathophysiology and management of low high-density lipoprotein cholesterol. Am J Cardiol. 1999;83(9B):22F-24F.
52. Buchwald H, Estok R, Fahrbach K, et al. Weight and type 2 diabetes after bariatric surgery: systematic review and meta-analysis. Am J Med. 2009;122:248e56.e5.
53. Schauer PR, Bhatt DL, Kirwan JP, et al. Bariatric surgery versus intensive medical therapy for diabetes 3-year outcomes. N Engl J Med. 2014;370:2002e13.

14

CHAPTER

Hypertension and Diabetes Mellitus

Medha Joshi, Romesh Khardori

INTRODUCTION

Hypertension affects approximately 50% of patients with diabetes. The prevalence of hypertension and diabetes is growing worldwide with increase in obesity and aging population. Both diabetes and hypertension are independent risk factors for atherosclerotic cardiovascular disease (ASCVD), heart failure and microvascular complications such as chronic kidney disease (CKD). Together, they have significant impact on morbidity and well as mortality. Therefore, it is extremely important to address blood pressure (BP) elevation in patients with diabetes.

Hypertension is defined as sustained BP elevation ≥140/90 mm Hg.[1] Elevated BP should be confirmed on a separate day. BP should be measured at every clinic visit after 5 minutes of rest in a seated position, with feet on the floor and arm supported at the heart level. Appropriate cuff size for the upper arm circumference should be used. Postural drop in BP could indicate autonomic neuropathy, therefore, orthostatic BP should be checked during initial visit and later as clinically indicated. Postural change in BP should be measured with patient standing unsupported at least for 2 minutes. It is important to measure heart rate simultaneously both while seated and after standing.

PATHOPHYSIOLOGY

The cause of hypertension in patients with diabetes is multifactorial. Obesity and insulin resistance have a major role to play. Hyperinsulinemia plays an important role in the pathophysiology and is also an independent risk factor for cardiovascular disease in patients with diabetes. Diabetic nephropathy is an important factor involved in the development of hypertension in patients with diabetes with increased peripheral vascular resistance being the hallmark for hypertension.[2] The involvement of renin-angiotensin-aldosterone system, adrenergic system, and calcium-calmodulin pathway are some additional proposed mechanisms. A longer duration of diabetes has been linked to arterial stiffness, increased sympathetic tone, abnormal vasomotor function, and changes in pulse pressure, which can also result in loss of usual nocturnal BP dip (nondippers). Nondipping may herald onset of manifest renal dysfunction such as proteinuria.

Majority of adults with high BP have primary hypertension (erroneously called essential-hypertension), the cause of which is not clearly known although genetic, and environmental factors such as excessive salt intake, obesity and sedentary lifestyle are thought to contribute. With increasing age, systolic blood pressure (SBP) tends to increase reflecting progressive stiffening of arterial circulation, which further accentuates ASCVD risk and CKD progression.[3] Hypertension is particularly common finding in people of African descent. It tends to occur at a younger age and is often more severe compared with non-African population.[4]

Secondary hypertension occurs in about 5% of all patients with hypertension where the cause can be identified and sometimes treated such as CKD, renal artery stenosis, obstructive sleep apnea and pheochromocytoma.[1] In patients with diabetes and hypertension when clinically indicated, endocrine workup to rule out thyroid dysfunction (hypothyroidism or hyperthyroidism), Cushing's syndrome and acromegaly should be considered (where phenotypic features exist or the index of suspicion is high). Lately primary aldosteronism has gained lot of press. It must be addressed in people deemed to have resistant hypertension.[1a]

BLOOD PRESSURE TARGETS AND MONITORING

The target or goal BP in patients with diabetes is debatable with varying recommendations from different societies. Guidelines from JNC 8 (Joint National Committee's eighth report) published in 2014 recommend a target SBP ≤140 mm Hg and diastolic blood pressure (DBP) ≤90 mm Hg. The American Diabetes Association (ADA)[5] recommends target SBP ≤140 mm Hg and DBP ≤80 mm Hg in patients without proteinuria, and a lower target SBP ≤130 mm Hg and DBP ≤80 mm Hg in those with proteinuria. Individualized treatment approach is recommended to account for any risks associated with significant BP reductions. In 2013 National Heart Lung and Blood Institute (NHLBI) announced that after JNC 8 no guidelines will be developed and that each society must develop its own guidelines.

For patients with higher cardiovascular risk (10-year ASCVD risk ≥15%) BP target of <130/80 mm Hg is considered appropriate, if safely attainable. Intensive BP control can lead to potential adverse effects such as orthostatic hypotension, syncope, falls, electrolyte abnormalities and acute kidney injury. Elderly frail patients and those with CKD are particularly at risk.[6] For individuals at lower cardiovascular risk (10-year ASCVD risk <15%) BP target of <140/90 mm Hg is reasonable.

Self-monitoring of BP at home should be encouraged in every patient with elevated BP. When discrepancies between office and home BP are noted, 24-hour ambulatory BP monitoring could be helpful to provide evidence of white coat hypertension and masked hypertension. Home BP monitoring may improve patient medication compliance and help reduce cardiovascular risk.[7] It should be noted that white coat hypertension is an example of labile hypertension, and hence not a totally inert entity.

LIFESTYLE MODIFICATION

It is essential to start lifestyle interventions early in management of both diabetes and mildly elevated BP (systolic >120 mm Hg or diastolic >80 mm Hg). Even moderate weight loss in overweight or obese patients is helpful in controlling hypertension, diabetes, and dyslipidemia. Increasing activity level and regular aerobic exercise should be recommended to all patients.[8]

Dietary Approaches to Stop Hypertension (DASH)-style eating pattern should be recommended for reduction of BP and need for medications. Sodium restriction (<2,300 mg/day) is important. Patients should be educated about the high salt content in foods such as canned foods, fast foods, chips, processed meat, pickles, soups, and bread. Other dietary interventions include caloric restriction, addition of fruits and vegetables (8–10 servings per day) and avoiding excessive alcohol consumption (no more than two servings per day in men and no more than one serving per day in women).[9]

Smoking cessation should be strongly encouraged at each office visit as smoking by itself is a major cardiovascular risk factor. Lifestyle management should be regarded as a compliment to drug therapy.

PHARMACOLOGIC MANAGEMENT

Patients with sustained BP elevation ≥140/90 confirmed in office setting should be promptly started on pharmacological therapy, in addition to lifestyle modification to achieve BP goals.

Patient with BP ≥160/100 confirmed in the office should be started on two medications or single-pill combination of medications with the goal of effectively achieving adequate BP control. In general, multiple drug therapy is required to achieve BP target.

Patients should be followed at regular intervals to monitor response for therapy. It is important to evaluate adherence to antihypertensive therapy at each visit before escalation of treatment. Single-pill combination antihypertensive therapy is preferred as it has shown to improve medication compliance.[10] Since there is association between absences of nocturnal BP dipping and ASCVD risk, bedtime dosing is preferred to reduce cardiovascular events.[11] Furthermore, it is important to consider the fact that peripheral vascular resistance is at its maximum in early hours of morning.

Several pharmacologic classes of antihypertensives have shown to reduce cardiovascular events in patients with diabetes (**Table 14.1**). These include angiotensin-converting enzyme (ACE) inhibitors, angiotensin receptor blockers (ARB), dihydropyridine calcium channel blockers (CCB) and thiazide-like diuretics. Multiple factors need to be considered while choosing antihypertensive therapy such as patient's cardiovascular status, renal function, race, and socioeconomic factors as well as medication efficacy, safety profile and cost.

Angiotensin-converting enzyme inhibitors offer several advantages. They protect against progression of moderately increased albuminuria due to type 1 diabetes mellitus (T1DM) and type 2 diabetes mellitus (T2DM). They are generally well-tolerated except potential of causing dry cough (mostly in females). Plasma potassium concentration should be monitored in patients with underlying renal insufficiency or hyperkalemia.

Angiotensin II receptor blockers have similar benefits as is ACE inhibitor without causing cough (although reported sporadically).

Combination therapy of ACE inhibitor with ARB or direct renin inhibitor should be avoided given the lack of synergistic cardiovascular benefit and increased risk of adverse effects including hyperkalemia, acute kidney injury and syncope.[12]

Dihydropyridine calcium channel blockers are overall well tolerated and have mild side effects such as peripheral edema and constipation. In the ACCOMPLISH trial, the combination of ACE inhibitor and amlodipine provided better cardiovascular protection in patients with diabetes compared with combination of ACE inhibitor and low-dose hydrochlorothiazide.[13]

According to JNC 8 recommendations,[8] initial therapy for nonblack patients with diabetes should be either with thiazide-type diuretics, ACE inhibitors, ARBs, CCBs. For African descent patients without CKD, thiazide diuretics or CCBs are the preferred initial treatment classes. These recommendations are based on the results of ALLHAT (Antihypertensive and Lipid-Lowering Treatment to Prevent Heart Attack Trial)[14] published in 2002 which showed in African descent individuals there was

TABLE 14.1: Commonly used antihypertensives for management of hypertension and diabetes in the United States.

Drug class	Advantages	Disadvantages
Angiotensin-converting enzyme (ACE) inhibitors • Benazepril (Lotensin) 5–40 mg daily • Captopril 12.5–100 mg twice daily • Enalapril (Vasotec) 5 mg,10–40 mg • Lisinopril (Prinivil, Zestril) 5–40 mg daily • Quinapril (Accupril) 10–80 mg daily • Ramipril (Altace) 2.5–20 mg daily	Decreases proteinuria and preserves renal function. Mortality benefit in heart failure	Not as effective in black population per ALLHAT. Side effects: Dry cough, angioedema
Angiotensin II antagonists [Angiotensin receptor blockers (ARB)] • Candesartan (Atacand) 8–32 mg daily Losartan (Cozaar) 25–100 mg daily • Olmesartan (Benicar) 20–40 mg daily • Telmisartan (Micardis) 20–80 mg daily • Valsartan (Diovan) 80–320 mg divided in 1–2 doses	Decreases proteinuria and preserves renal function. Mortality benefit in heart failure Well tolerated No cough	Side effects: Hyperkalemia, mild creatinine increase. Angioedema is rare
Calcium channel blocker (CCB)—Dihydropyridine • Amlodipine (Norvasc) 2.5–10 mg daily • Nicardipine SR (Cardene SR) 60–120 mg divided in 2 doses Nifedipine long-acting (Adalat CC, Procardia XL) 30–60 mg daily	Equally effective in all racial and ethnic groups	Side effects: Peripheral edema, constipation
Thiazide diuretic • Chlorothiazide (Diuril) 500–2,000 mg daily divided in 1–2 doses • Chlorthalidone (generic) 6.25–25 mg daily • Hydrochlorothiazide (Microzide) 12.5–50 mg daily	Potent. Especially effective in black population with salt sensitive hypertension	Side effects: Hypokalemia, hyperglycemia, hyponatremia, and hyperuricemia

significant reduction in BP and cardiovascular events when treated with thiazides compared with ACE inhibitors.

In patients with CKD according to JNC 8 recommendations, ACE inhibitors or ARBs are the preferred initial therapeutic classes given their ability to reduce progression of kidney disease.[15] These agents are prescribed irrespective of ethnic background. Additionally, since proteinuria independently predicts worse renal outcome several guidelines suggest tighter BP control in patients with proteinuria. ACE inhibitor or ARB is recommended first-line treatment for hypertension in patients with diabetes and significant albuminuria (albumin to creatinine ratio ≥300 mg/g) and should be considered in those with albumin to creatinine ratio 30–299 mg/g. It is our position that microalbuminuria being a major predictor of progression of renal disease has been overstated.

Patients with advanced CKD [estimated glomerular filtration rate (eGFR) <45 mL/min/1.73 m^2] are at risk for developing hyperkalemia. Monitoring of serum potassium, creatinine and eGFR should be performed at least annually in all patients treated with ACE inhibitors, ARBs and diuretics and mineralocorticoid receptor antagonist.

In patients without albuminuria, the risk of progression of CKD is low, therefore there is no additional benefit of ACE inhibitor or ARB when compared with CCBs or thiazide-like diuretics.[16] It is our position that temptation must be avoided to label hospitalized patients as suffering from CKD based on indices (eGFR and serum creatinine) obtained while patients are acutely sick. These indices must be rechecked in out-patient setting after patient has returned to basal health state.

Hypertension is a major risk factor for development of heart failure (HF), which could be with reduced ejection fraction (HFrEF) or with preserved ejection fraction (HFpEF).

In patients with HFrEF, medications such as ACE inhibitors, ARBs, beta blockers and mineralocorticoid receptor antagonists are all effective in improving clinical outcomes. Angiotensin receptor-neprilysin inhibitor (ARNI)-sacubitril-valsartan is indicated for the treatment of HFrEF as an alternative to ACE inhibitors or ARBs. Diuretics provide symptomatic improvement.[1]

In the ALLHAT there was lower rate of new onset heart failure in patients treated with low-dose thiazide compared with amlodipine and lisinopril. Treatment should be individualized after discussion of risk versus benefit of therapy with the patient.

Beta-blockers as an antihypertensive class have not shown to reduce mortality, except in patients with significant coronary artery disease (myocardial infarction and active angina) or HFrEF which should be the primary indications for prescribing these medications.[17]

Resistant hypertension is defined as BP >140/90 mm Hg in a patient treated with three or more antihypertensive medications, at least one of which is a diuretic. It is important to rule out other causes for uncontrolled hypertension (pseudo-resistance) such as medication nonadherence, suboptimal antihypertensive therapy, white coat effect and poor BP measurement technique and substance/drug induced hypertension before labeling resistant hypertension. Workup for secondary hypertension should be performed in patients with resistant hypertension. Mineralocorticoid receptor antagonists are effective for management of resistant hypertension in patients with T2DM when added to existing treatment with an ACE inhibitor or ARB, thiazide-like diuretic, and CCBs. They have additional cardiovascular benefits and decrease albuminuria as well.[18]

GLUCOSE LOWERING THERAPIES (AMERICAN DIABETES ASSOCIATION)

Given concerns for increased cardiovascular risk in patients with T2DM, in 2008 United States Food and Drug Administration (FDA) issued guidance to drug industry to perform cardiovascular outcomes trials for all new medications.[19] Since then, two classes of glucose lowering therapies have emerged based on randomized controlled trials supporting their evidence for cardiovascular risk reduction.

Glucagon-like peptide 1 (GLP-1) receptor agonists and sodium-glucose cotransporter-2 (SGLT-2) inhibitors are currently the preferred glucose lowering agents in patients with T2DM and established ASCVD or CKD.

Majority of patients with T2DM are overweight or obese. GLP-1 receptor agonists help with weight reduction, which is an added advantage of this class of medication. Four GLP-1 receptor agonists (Liraglutide, Albiglutide, Semaglutide, and Dulaglutide) have been FDA approved as agents to reduce ASCVD risk.

Approximately 50% of patients with T2DM may develop heart failure,[20] many of which have coexistent hypertension. Three FDA approved SGLT-2 inhibitors (Canagliflozin, Empagliflozin, Dapagliflozin) have shown to reduce the incidence of heart failure, adverse cardiovascular events, and heart failure hospitalization while providing renal protection with CKD, ADA. Heart failure in type-2 diabetic patient increases the risk of mortality. Therefore, role of SGLT-2 inhibitor therapy cannot be overemphasized. Recently approved another SGLT-2 inhibitor—Ertugliflozin did not fare well against placebo. A combination of both cardiovascular death and hospitalization for heart failure occurred in about 8% and 9%, respectively.[21]

ATHEROSCLEROTIC CARDIOVASCULAR DISEASE PREVENTION

Atherosclerotic cardiovascular disease includes coronary artery disease, cerebrovascular disease, or peripheral artery disease. It is the leading cause of morbidity and mortality in people with diabetes, the risk of which increases with coexistent hypertension.

The 10-year ASCVD risk calculator by the American College of Cardiology/American Heart Association is a widely used tool to estimate 10-year ASCVD. The calculator (available online at tools.acc.org/ASCVD-Risk-Estimator-Plus) includes diabetes and hypertension as risk factors and helps to guide therapy based on risk stratification.[22]

Statin therapy is the treatment of choice for low-density lipoprotein (LDL) reduction and is recommended for primary prevention of ASCVD in patients with diabetes aged 40–75 years. For younger patients with diabetes aged 20–39 years with an additional ASCVD risk factor (which includes hypertension) it may be reasonable to initiate statin therapy. In patients with diabetes and 10 year ASCVD risk >20%, addition of ezetimibe to maximally tolerated statin therapy is recommended to reduce LDL-C by 50% ADA. Statins are contraindicated in pregnancy, therefore it should be cautiously prescribed in females of reproductive age group.

Aspirin therapy (75–162 mg/day) could be used for primary prevention in both men and women after age 50 years with diabetes and at least one major additional risk factor (which includes hypertension, family history of premature ASCVD, dyslipidemia, smoking, CKD/albuminuria). It should not be prescribed to patients who are at increased risk of bleeding such as older age, history of gastrointestinal bleeding, anemia, renal disease (ADA). A recent meta-regression analysis did not find support role for primary prevention of ASCVD in high risk patients.[23]

PREGNANCY CONSIDERATIONS

Hypertensive disorders of pregnancy are one of the leading causes of maternal and perinatal mortality worldwide, and are classified as:

- Pre-existing (chronic) hypertension.
- Gestational hypertension (developing ≥20 weeks' gestation).
- Preeclampsia (gestational hypertension with new proteinuria or adverse conditions affecting an organ system such as central nervous system, cardiorespiratory, renal, hepatic, hematological or fetal placental unit.

- Preeclampsia superimposed on chronic hypertension. Preeclampsia rates have significantly increased by 25% between 1987 and 2004. Women with chronic hypertension and T1DM or T2DM are at high risk for developing preeclampsia and therefore, they should receive low-dose aspirin 81 mg/day for preeclampsia prophylaxis initiated between 12 and 28 weeks of gestation and continued until delivery.[24]

  In pregnant patients with diabetes who have pre-existing hypertension, a BP target of ≤135/85 mm Hg is recommended with the goal of reducing maternal and fetal complications.[25] According to the CHIPS (Control of hypertension in Pregnancy Study) performed in pregnant women with chronic hypertension, targeting BP <135/85 was associated with reduce likelihood of maternal accelerated hypertension and no demonstrable adverse fetal outcome.
- Methyldopa, labetalol and long acting nifedipine are the preferred antihypertensive agents known to be safe and effective during pregnancy.[26] ACE inhibitors, ARBs and spironolactone are contraindicated during pregnancy due to risk of fetal damage. Diuretics are generally not recommended for BP control but may be used later during pregnancy for volume management. After delivery, patients with elevated BP should be observed in the hospital for 72 hours and closely monitored in the postpartum period. Long-term follow-up is recommended given increase lifetime cardiovascular risk.

SUMMARY

Hypertension in patients with diabetes must be addressed like any other situation where diabetes mellitus does not coexist. Correction of obesity and sleep apnea would have huge benefit. There is growing evidence that BP lowering with antihypertensive drugs is significantly associated with lower risk of incident dementia or cognitive impairment.[27]

All cause death is similar for first-line RAS inhibitors, first-line calcium channel blockers, thiazides and beta-blockers. There are differences for some morbidity outcomes, however.

Judicious use of SGLT-2 inhibitors may be considered in those patients whose hypertension is complicated by heart failure. However, not all SGLT-2 inhibitors are created equal when it comes to effect on heart failure.

Often questions arise about use of hormonal contraception in young women with coexisting medical conditions we recommend reference to American College of Obstetrics and Gynecology Bulletin # 206.[28]

REFERENCES

1. Unger T, Borghi C, Charchar F, Khan NA, Poulter NR, Prabhakaran D, et al. International Society of Hypertension Global Hypertension Practice Guidelines 2020. Hypertension. 2020;75:1334-57.

1a. Brown J. Siddiqui M, Calhoun DA, et al. The Unrecognized Prevalence of Primary Aldosteronism: A Cross-sectional Study. Ann Intern Med. 2020;173: 10-20.

2. Epstein M, Sowers JR. Diabetes mellitus and hypertension. Hypertension. 1992;19(5):403-18.
3. Weber MA, Schiffrin EL, White WB, Mann S, Lindholm LH, Kenerson JG, et al. Clinical practice guidelines for the management of hypertension in the community a statement by the American Society of Hypertension and the International Society of Hypertension. J Hypertens. 2014;32:3-15.
4. Carson AP, Howard G, Burke GL, Shea S, Levitan EB, Muntner P. Ethnic differences in hypertension incidence among middle-aged and older adults: the multiethnic study of atherosclerosis. Hypertension. 2011;57(6):1101-7.
5. American Diabetes Association. 10. Cardiovascular Disease and Risk Management: Standards of Medical Care in Diabetes-2020. Diabetes Care. 2020;43(Suppl 1):S111-1340.
6. Sink KM, Evans GW, Shorr RI, Bates JT, Berlowitz D, Conroy MB, et al. Syncope, hypotension, and falls in the treatment of hypertension: results from the randomized clinical systolic blood pressure intervention trial. J Am Geriatr Soc. 2018;66:679-86.
7. Sega R, Facchetti R, and Bombelli M, Cesana G, Corrao G, Grassi G, et al. Prognostic value of ambulatory and home blood pressures compared with office blood pressure in the general population: follow-up results from the Pressioni Arteriose Monitoratee Loro Associazioni (PAMELA) study. Circulation. 2005;111:1777-83.
8. James PA, Oparil S, Carter BL, Cushman WC, Dennison-Himmelfarb C, Handler J, et al. 2014 evidence-based guideline for the management of high blood pressure in adults: report from the panel members appointed to the Eighth Joint National Committee (JNC 8). JAMA. 2014;311:507-20.
9. Sacks FM, Svetkey LP, Vollmer WM, Appel LJ, Bray GA, Harsha D, et al. DASH-Sodium Collaborative Research Group. Effects on blood pressure of reduced dietary sodium and the Dietary Approaches to Stop Hypertension (DASH) diet. N Engl J Med. 2001;344:3-10.
10. Bangalore S, Kamalakkannan G, Parkar S, Messerli FH. Fixed-dose combinations improve medication compliance: a meta-analysis. Am J Med. 2007;120(8):713-9.
11. Zhao P, Xu P, Wan C, Wang Z. Evening versus morning dosing regimen drug therapy for hypertension. Cochrane Database Syst Rev. 2011;10:CD004184.
12. Fried LF, Emanuele N, Zhang JH, Brophy M, Conner TA, Duckworth W, et al. VA NEPHRON-D Investigators. Combined angiotensin inhibition for the treatment of diabetic nephropathy. N Engl J Med. 2013;369:1892-903.
13. Weber MA, Bakris GL, Jamerson K, Weir M, Kjeldsen SE, Devereux RB, et al. ACCOMPLISH Investigators. Cardiovascular events during differing hypertension therapies in patients with diabetes. J Am Coll Cardiol. 2010;56:77-85.
14. ALLHAT Officers and Coordinators for the ALLHAT Collaborative Research Group. Major outcomes in high-risk hypertensive patients randomized to angiotensin-converting enzyme inhibitor or calcium channel blocker vs diuretic: the Antihypertensive and Lipid-Lowering Treatment to Prevent Heart Attack Trial (ALLHAT). JAMA. 2002;288(23):2981-97.
15. de Boer IH, Bangalore S, Benetos A, Davis AM, Michos ED, Muntner P, et al. Diabetes and hypertension: a position statement by the American Diabetes Association. Diabetes Care. 2017;40:1273-84.

16. Bangalore S, Fakheri R, Toklu B, Messerli FH. Diabetes mellitus as a compelling indication for use of renin angiotensin system blockers: systematic review and meta-analysis of randomized trials. BMJ. 2016;352:i438.
17. Ettehad D, Emdin CA, Kiran A, Anderson SG, Callender T, Emberson J, et al. Blood pressure lowering for prevention of cardiovascular disease and death: a systematic review and meta-analysis. Lancet. 2016;387(10022):957-67.
18. Williams B, MacDonald TM, Morant S, Webb DJ, Sever P, McInnes G, et al. British Hypertension Society's PATHWAY Studies Group. Spironolactone versus placebo, bisoprolol, and doxazosin to determine the optimal treatment for drug-resistant hypertension (PATHWAY-2): a randomised, double-blind, crossover trial. Lancet. 2015;386:2059-68.
19. US Food and Drug Administration. Guidance for industry. Diabetes mellitus—evaluating cardiovascular risk in new antidiabetic therapies to treat type 2 diabetes. Silver Spring. MD, 2008.
20. Kannel WB, Hjortland M, Castelli WP. Role of diabetes in congestive heart failure: the Framingham study. Am J Cardiol. 1974;34:29-34.
21. Cannon CP, Pratley R, Dagogo-Jack S, Mancuso J, Huyck S, Masiukiewicz U, et al. Cardiovascular Outcomes with Ertugliflozin in Type2 Diabetes. N Engl J Med. 2020.
22. Grundy SM, Stone NJ, Bailey AL, Beam C, Birtcher KK, Blumenthal RS, et al. 2018. AHA/ACC/AACVPR/AAPA/ABC/ACPM/ADA/AGS/APhA/ASPC/NLA/PCNA Guideline on the management of blood cholesterol: executive summary: a report of the American College of Cardiology/American Heart Association Task Force on Clinical Practice Guidelines. J Am Coll Cardiol. 2019;73:3168-209.
23. Nudy M, Cooper J, Ghahramani M, Ruzieh M, Mandrola J, Foy AJ. Aspirin for Primary Atherosclerotic Cardiovascular Disease Prevention as Baseline Risk Increases: A Meta-Regression Analysis. Am J Med. 2020;133:1056.
24. Gestational hypertension and preeclampsia. Obstet Gynecol. 2020;135(6): e237-60.
25. Magee LA, von Dadelszen P, Rey E, Ross S, Asztalos E, Murphy KE, et al. Less-tight versus tight control of hypertension in pregnancy. N Engl J Med. 2015;372:407-17.
26. Hypertension in pregnancy: executive summary. Obstet Gynecol. 2013;122(5): 1122-31.
27. Hughes D, Judge C, Murphy R, Loughlin E, Costello M, Whiteley W, et al. Association of blood pressure lowering with incident dementia or cognitive impairment: a systematic review and meta-analysis. JAMA. 2020;323(19):1934.
28. ACOG Practice Bulletin No 206: Use of hormonal contraception in woman with coexisting medical conditions. Obstet and Gynecol. 2019;133(2):e128.

15
CHAPTER

Diabetes in the Elderly

Anju Agarwal, Ved V Gossain

INTRODUCTION

Globally, approximately 463 million (about 9%) adults (20–79 years) were living with diabetes in 2019. This number is expected to increase to 700 million by the year 2045. Almost half the people (232 million) people with diabetes are undiagnosed.[1]

The US has one of the highest rates of prevalence of diabetes (10.5%) followed closely by the prevalence in India (10.4%).[2]

The percentage of adults with diabetes increases with age reaching 26.8% among those 65 years or older.[3] Moreover, the percentage of people older than 65 years is increasing worldwide. In the USA, the number of Americans aged 65 years and older is expected to increase from 16% in 2018 to 22% in 2050.[4] The diabetes in the elderly therefore, appears to be a major health problem.

Among older adults with diabetes, >90% have type 2 diabetes mellitus (T2DM), although some people with type 1 diabetes mellitus (T1DM) are living into the elderly age group. The incidence of newly diagnosed diabetes is found to be highest in the individuals in the age group of 65–79 years, which is nearly 8.8%. While about half of the individuals with diabetes between the age 60 and 69 years report that they have had the disease for duration of >10 years, about 20% of the patients above 80 years of age report that duration of disease was <5 years.[5]

PATHOPHYSIOLOGY OF HYPERGLYCEMIA IN THE ELDERLY

Type 2 diabetes mellitus occurs in the older population as a result of a complex interaction among genetic, lifestyle, and aging influences (**Flowchart 15.1**).

The lifestyle changes may include impaired mobility and the changes in body composition, namely increased adipose

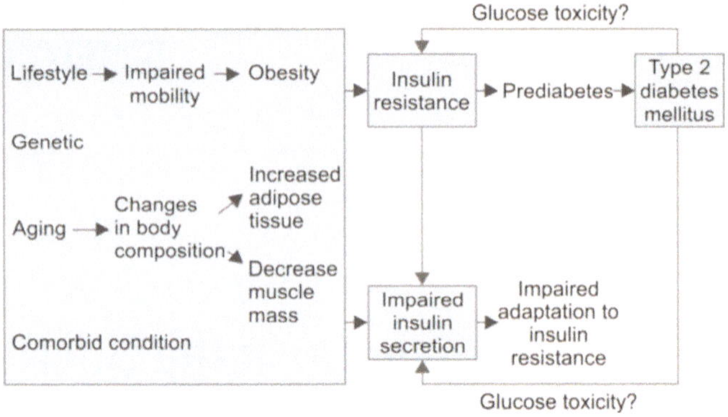

FLOWCHART 15.1: Model for age-related hyperglycemia.

Source: Adapted from Chang AM, Halter JB. Aging and insulin secretion. Am J Physiol Endocrinol Metab. 2003;284:E7-12.

tissue and a decrease in muscle mass further increase insulin resistance.[6] Chronic exposure to hyperglycemia can lead to glucose toxicity, which can further result in worsening of the insulin resistance and impairment of pancreatic β-cell function. Lipotoxicity due to exposure to products of fat cell lipolysis can also result in this vicious cycle, similar to visceral obesity as well as intramyocellular fat. In an individual or family, the heterogeneity of T2DM possibly indicates the varying roles of several factors in the development of hyperglycemia. The knowledge of these factors can provide a basis for the glucose-lowering medications selection for an individual patient.

DIAGNOSIS OF DIABETES IN THE ELDERLY

The criteria for the diagnosis of diabetes are same as they are in younger individuals and are listed below in **Table 15.1**.

In the absence of unequivocal hyperglycemia, diagnosis requires two abnormal test results from the same sample or in two separate samples.

The Endocrine Society recommends obtaining a 2-hour glucose postoral glucose tolerance test measurement for patients of age ≥65 years without known diabetes and meeting criteria for prediabetes by glycated hemoglobin (HbA1c) or fasting plasma glucose. As recommended by the Endocrine Society, in selected cases, such screening should be repeated every 2 years.[7] This recommendation applies in particular to high-risk population that includes first-degree relative with diabetes, overweight or obese, sleep apnea, high-risk race or ethnicity (such as Latino, African-American, Asian-American, Native American, and Pacific Islander), physical inactivity, hypertension (≥140/90 mm Hg

TABLE 15.1: Criteria for diagnosis of diabetes and prediabetes.

Tests	Normal	Prediabetes	Diabetes
Fasting plasma glucose*	<100 mg/dL (<5.6 mmol/L)	100–125 mg/dL (5.6–5.9 mmol/L)	≥126 mg/dL (≥7 mmol/L)
2-hour postglucose**	<140 mg/dL (<7.8 mmol/L)	140–199 mg/dL (7.8–11.0 mmol/L)	≥200 mg/dL (≥11.1 mmol/L)
HbA1c***	<5.5%	5.5–6.4%	≥6.5%
Random plasma glucose	–	–	≥200 + symptoms of diabetes

*After at least 8 hours of no caloric intake.

**After a 75-g glucose load.

***The test should be performed in a laboratory using a method that is National Glycohemoglobin Standardization Program certified and standardized to the Diabetes Control and Complications Trial assay.

(HbA1c: glycosylated hemoglobin)

Source: Adapted from American Diabetes Association. 2. Classification and Diagnosis of Diabetes: Standards of Medical Care in Diabetes-2020. Diabetes Care. 2020;43:S14-31.

or on treatment for hypertension), high-density lipoprotein cholesterol level <35 mg/dL (0.90 mmol/L), prior history of cardiovascular disease (CVD), and/or a triglyceride level >250 mg/dL (2.82 mmol/L).[7] However, for patients who have limited life expectancy, this recommendation is not appropriate.

COMPLICATIONS OF DIABETES

Chronic complications of diabetes typically develop in people with long duration of diabetes. However, it cannot be assumed that the elderly are somehow protected because they may not have the duration of diabetes long enough to result in complications. On the contrary, the incidence of stroke, ischemic heart disease, and congestive heart failure is significantly higher in the elderly compared to the younger population unrelated to diabetes itself.

The dramatic effect of age on the incidence of major diabetes complications is illustrated in **Figure 15.1**.

Diabetic nephropathy is present in nearly 50% of diabetic patients of age >65 years. Diabetic nephropathy manifests as impairment in glomerular filtration rate (GFR), albuminuria, or both. The rate is found to be highest in the individuals of age 75 years or more. In old age people with diabetes, the risk for lower extremity amputation is reported to be 10-fold higher as compared to those without diabetes.[8] So, for the care of old age patients with diabetes, measures should be prevention and treatment of these complications.

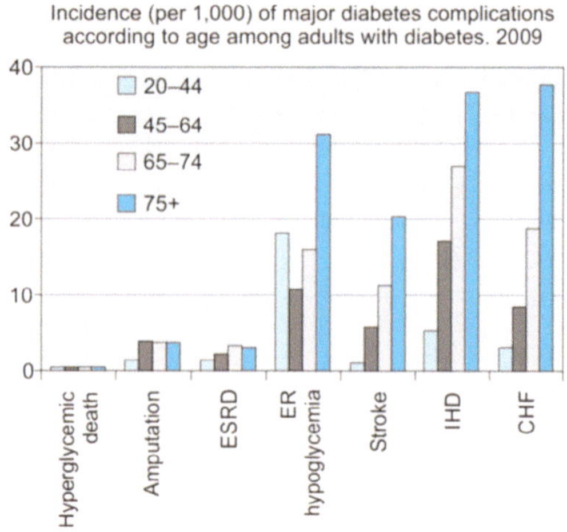

(CHF: congestive heart failure; ER: emergency room; ESRD: end-stage renal disease; IHD: ischemic heart disease)

FIG. 15.1: Incidence (per 1,000) of major diabetes complications according to age among adults with diabetes, 2009.

Source: Reproduced from Centers for Disease Control and Prevention (CDC). (2019). Diabetes Data and Statistics. [online] Available from https://www.cdc.gov/diabetes/data/index.html. [Last accessed April, 2020].

MANAGEMENT OF PREDIABETES AND DIABETES IN THE ELDERLY

Approximately 34.5% of all US adults had prediabetes based on their fasting glucose or HbA1c levels whereas 10.5% adults had prediabetes based on both elevated fasting glucose and HbA1c levels.[3]

The risk for cardiovascular complications appears to be increased both in prediabetes and diabetes.[9,10]

Prediabetes progresses to diabetes at approximately 5% per year if there are no interventions.[11,12] Several studies have also shown that the rate of progression to diabetes can be slowed by lifestyle interventions or medications.[13] In the Diabetes Prevention Program, in people over the age of 60 years, lifestyle intervention of increased physical activity to reduce body weight, reduced the rate of progression to diabetes by 71% during 4 years as compared to a relative risk reduction of 59% in the age group 45–59 years and 48% in the age group 25–44 years.[14] The reduced rate of progression to diabetes was maintained during 15 years of follow-up and metformin was less effective as compared to the lifestyle modification in this age group.[15] A recent meta-analysis involving 5,000 subjects confirmed these findings.[16] For these reasons, screening for diabetes and prediabetes is recommended in subjects over the age of 65 years, using either fasting plasma glucose or HbA1c.

TREATMENT OF DIABETES

The treatment plan must be individualized through a shared decision process. Sometimes, there may be a discrepancy in the goals of treatment from the physician's perspective and those from the patient's perspective. For example, common goals of physicians treating diabetes include alleviation of symptoms, reverse the metabolic effects of hyperglycemia (glucose toxicity), and to prevent the long-term complications of diabetes. On the other hand, in a small study of older patients with diabetes, 43% reported independence in activities of daily living (ADL) as their goal, 29% reported to be alive and healthy as their goal, and 14% reported weight loss as their goal. Less than 3.5% subjects reported adherence to diet, exercise or medication, avoidance of symptoms, and control of blood sugar as their goal.[17] With a detailed discussion, a treatment plan should be mutually agreed upon. In 50% cases, medical experience of family and friends and in 43% cases, experience with healthcare professionals shaped patient's goals.[17] Involving significant other family members in the decision process may also improve adherence. Similarly, the healthcare team should decide who will be the physician in charge of the care, the endocrinology consultant, or the patient's primary care physician or will the case be managed jointly.[7]

In the care of older adults with diabetes, assessment of the overall health status is important because besides diabetes many other factors affect the functional status of patients. There are many other geriatric syndromes that are common in the older population including depression, cognitive impairment and urinary incontinence especially in women, alcohol abuse, polypharmacy, injurious falls, and persistent pain.[18]

It is recommended that older adults with diabetes should undergo a screening for cognitive impairment or dementia at the initial visit and annually as appropriate. Blood pressure and body mass index (BMI) measurement should also be included in the overall assessment. Additional laboratory tests may include electrocardiogram (ECG), lipid panel, bone mineral density, and screening for abdominal aortic aneurysm (AAA) in selected cases.[19]

According to the recommendations of the United States Preventive Services Task Force (USPSTF), one time screening for AAA along with ultrasonography should be done for men who have ever smoked; it also recommends against routine screening for AAA for women who have never smoked as well as lack a family history of AAA.[20] Diabetes-specific assessment should include an assessment of chronic complications (retinopathy, nephropathy, and neuropathy) because they may affect the quality of life and overall survival.

LIFESTYLE MANAGEMENT

Nutrition

Several old age adults who have T2DM are overweight or obese. The age-related decline in physical function is exacerbated by obesity and it also leads to frailty in old age adults. In these adults, the appropriate treatment is still in controversy. Advice of weight loss is typically given to the young age adults having prediabetes or diabetes; however, in the old age population, therapies for aggressive weight loss are not recommended.

A strategy of a combination of diet, physical activity, and behavior therapy to achieve and maintain a weight loss of about 5% can be recommended for overweight or obese adults.[21]

Diabetes in older adults is often associated with reduced muscle mass and strength resulting in sarcopenia.[22,23] Diabetes is also recognized as a risk factor for frailty, which is characterized by decline in physical performance and increased risk of poor health. The management of frailty, therefore, includes adequate caloric and protein intake along with an exercise program.[24]

According to the American Diabetes Association, the goals of the nutrition therapy for people with diabetes are:[25]

- Improving overall health and particularly improving blood pressure, HbA1c, and cholesterol levels; there are different goals for individuals depending on age, health history, present health conditions, and duration of diabetes.
- Addressing individual nutrition requirements on the basis of accessibility of healthy food options, personal and cultural preferences, willingness and capability of making behavioral changes, health literacy and numeracy, and hurdles to change.
- Promoting and supporting healthy eating habits, focusing on a range of nutrient-rich foods in proper portion sizes.
- Preserving the enjoyment of eating by supplying optimistic messages about food options available, thus limiting food options only in case it is indicated by scientific evidences.
- Achieving and maintaining the body weight goals.
- Delaying or preventing complications associated with diabetes.
- Providing practical tools for day-to-day meal planning for diabetic patient.

It is apparent that there is no such thing as an "American Diabetes Association diet" and that one size does not fit all. The dietary prescription must be individualized. The estimated daily calorie needs for older adults based on age, sex, and physical activity are summarized below in **Table 15.2**.

Although several studies have attempted to determine the best mixture of macronutrients, an ideal mixture has not emerged. Most patients with diabetes also consume approximately the same mixture of macronutrient as the

TABLE 15.2: Estimated calorie needs per day for older adults by age, sex, and physical activity level.

Males				Females		
Age (years)	Sedentary*	Mod active**	Active***	Sedentary	Mod active	Active
61–65	2,000	2,400	2,600	1,600	1,800	2,000
66–70	2,000	2,200	2,600	1,600	1,800	2,000
71–75	2,000	2,200	2,600	1,600	1,800	2,000
76 and up	2,000	2,200	2,400	1,600	1,800	2,000

*Sedentary means a lifestyle that includes only the physical activity of daily living.

**Mod active = Moderately active means a lifestyle that includes physical activity equivalent to walking 1.5–3 miles/day at 3–4 miles/h in addition to the activities of independent living.

***Active means a lifestyle that includes walking >3 miles/day at 3–4 miles/h in addition to the activities of independent living.

Source: Institute of Medicine. Dietary Reference Intakes for Energy, Carbohydrate, Fiber, Fat, Fatty Acids, Cholesterol, Protein, and Amino acids. Washington: The National Academic Press; 2002.

general public. Approximately 45% of calories are obtained from carbohydrates, 36–40% calories from fat, and the remainder 16–18% from proteins. Individualization of macronutrients should also be based on the need for the degree of control of hyperglycemia, physical activity, food preference, and the availability of food.[25]

Aging itself is associated with several factors that may affect the food selection and preparation which may limit the food intake. These include difficulties in shopping for food, limited cooking facilities, declining chemosensory perception (decreased sense of taste and smell), loss of appetite, poor dentition, and physical disabilities such as arthritis, difficulty with swallowing, loneliness, bereavement, and limited disposable income.[26]

A prospective study of Mediterranean diet including subjects over the age of 60 years obtained detailed dietary histories and calculated the Mediterranean diet score. The study concluded that a 2-unit increment in the diet score was associated with 8% (3–12%) reduction in mortality.[27] A consideration to the Mediterranean diet should therefore, be given if acceptable to the patients.

Exercise

For most adults, 30 minutes of moderate exertion (walking, stair climbing) and strength training are recommended.[28] However, for older adults, the exercise prescription should be modified based on individual circumstances. Any amount of exercise is better than being sedentary even if the health status of the person prevents a person from achieving the recommended targets. Physical activity decreases the risk of chronic disease, resistance training preserves muscle strength, and flexibility exercises improve and maintain range of movement of joints.[29]

Individualized prescription including all these components should be provided. Many community resources are available to help older adults lead a healthy lifestyle and should be utilized. In addition, it should be ensured that subjects get at least 6–8 hours of sleep because inadequate sleep leads to obesity and frailty. Advice should also be provided for stopping smoking and alcohol consumption in moderation (up to two drinks a day for men and one drink a day for women).

CONTROL OF DIABETES

The level of control of hyperglycemia should be individualized. In otherwise healthy adults, with few or no coexisting chronic illnesses and good cognitive function as well as good functional status, an HbA1c target of <7.5% may be selected.[19] On the other hand, adults with multiple comorbidities and impaired functional status, an HbA1c target of 8% or 8.5% may be selected. However, symptomatic hyperglycemia should be avoided. An HbA1c of 8.5% approximately correlates to a glucose level of 200 mg/dL. Higher HbA1c targets may result in hyperglycemia with symptoms.

HYPOGLYCEMIA

Patients should be carefully monitored and hypoglycemia should be avoided. In the elderly individuals, it may be difficult to diagnose hypoglycemia as the symptoms associated with hypoglycemia are less specific. It has been reported that with the advancement of age, cognitive decline was associated with enhanced risk of hypoglycemia; on the other hand, severe hypoglycemia was reported to be associated with dementia.[30]

Severe hypoglycemia may result in serious vascular events such as acute cardiac failure, myocardial infarction, ventricular arrhythmias, and stroke.[31-33]

PHARMACOLOGICAL TREATMENT OF DIABETES IN THE ELDERLY

For patients with T1DM, insulin is essential. Most patients would require long-acting insulin as the basal insulin and short-acting insulin to control the postprandial rise of glucose. The regimen however should be kept simple. If the patient has already been on an insulin pump, the pump therapy may be continued. However, introducing pump therapy at an advanced age may be difficult. Approximately, half the total dose of insulin can be given as the basal dose and the remainder as prandial dose in divide doses. Patients should be taught to adjust their dose of prandial insulin based on the anticipated carbohydrate intake and counting carbohydrates can therefore be quite helpful.[34]

For patients with T2DM, if the lifestyle intervention is not sufficient to achieve the glycemic targets, treatment with drugs should be introduced. Almost everyone agrees that metformin should be the first drug for the treatment of T2DM. It should be continued as long as it is tolerated and not contraindicated. Additional drugs can be introduced as needed. For that, a patient-centered approach should be used to guide the choice of other drugs that are added to metformin. If further lowering of glucose is needed, dipeptidyl peptidase-4 (DPP-4) inhibitors or glucagon-like peptide-1 (GLP-1) receptor agonists can be added in preference to adding insulin. For those with-high risk or established atherosclerotic cardiovascular disease (ASCVD), established renal disease, or heart failure, sodium-glucose cotransporter-2 (SGLT-2) inhibitors or GLP-1 receptor agonists with demonstrated cardiovascular benefit are recommended independent of HbA1c levels.[35] The pharmacologic details of drugs used in the management of diabetes are discussed in greater detail in the other chapters of this book.

MANAGEMENT OF RISK FACTORS

Management of Hypertension

Atherosclerotic cardiovascular disease, which includes coronary heart disease, cerebrovascular disease, and peripheral vascular disease, is the leading cause of morbidity and mortality for individuals with diabetes. Hypertension and increased low-density lipoprotein cholesterol (LDL-C) are clear risk factors for atherosclerotic heart disease and diabetes also is an independent risk factor.[36] Hypertension is not only a major risk factor of macrovascular disease, but it is also a risk factor for microvascular complications.

Blood pressure should be measured at each clinic visit. A diagnosis of hypertension defined as a blood pressure >140/90 mm Hg that should be confirmed after repeated measurements. Several studies have demonstrated that treatment of blood pressure to a level of <140/90 mm Hg reduces these complications.[37] Lower blood pressure targets have been evaluated in large randomized trials and meta-analysis, but taken together these studies indicate that treating blood pressure to a level of <140/90 mm Hg is beneficial. Lower targets may offer some additional benefits that appear to be less robust. Lower blood pressure targets may therefore, be appropriate in selected cases.[38]

Like the other aspects of the care of elderly individuals, blood pressure targets should also be individualized through shared decision-making. For most individuals, a blood pressure target of <140/90 mm Hg seems appropriate. In selected individuals with higher cardiovascular risk, a blood pressure target of <130/80 mm Hg may be appropriate if it can be safely achieved (further details of management of hypertension in diabetes, including the use of various drugs, are included in the Chapter 14: Management of Hypertension in Diabetes by Dr Khardori).

Management of Hyperlipidemia

Besides hypertension, hyperlipidemia is a major cardiovascular risk factor for ASCVD. Lifestyle modification including weight loss (if indicated, dietary modification and increased physical activity as tolerated) should be recommended to improve the lipid profile and reduce the risk of developing ASCVD in patients with diabetes.[36] For dietary modifications, Dietary Approaches to Stop Hypertension (DASH) or Mediterranean diets have been suggested.

The American College of Cardiology/American Heart Association guidelines[39] suggest that:

- In all individuals, a healthy lifestyle across the life course should be emphasized.
- In patients with ASCVD, LDL-C should be reduced by ≥50% with the use of high-intensity statin or maximally tolerated statin.
- In patients 40–75 years of age with diabetes mellitus and LDL ≥70 mg/dL, moderate-intensity statin therapy should be started without even calculating the 10-year ASCVD risk.

According to a systemic review for management of hyperlipidemia, it was reported that for primary prevention, the risk of coronary artery disease as well as myocardial infarction is decreased by the statins, but it did not reduced stroke or all-cause or cardiovascular mortality.[40]

For secondary prevention, statins decreased coronary artery disease, myocardial infarction, cardiovascular mortality, all-cause mortality, and revascularization. Intensive (as compared to less intensive) statin therapy decreased the risk of heart failure and coronary artery disease. In patients of age above 75 years, use of statins is less evident. According to a posthoc secondary data analysis of the ALLHAT-LLT (Antihypertensive and Lipid-lowering Treatment to Prevent Heart Attack) study that included patients of age 65 years or more, it was observed that on giving pravastatin for primary prevention to old age adults having hypertension and moderate hyperlipidemia, no benefit was noted.[41]

However, despite that the use of statins in persons older than 75 years has recently increased.[42] In most adults, the treatment of hypercholesterolemia generally would have started far before the age of 75–80 years. In that case, there is no need to discontinue statin due to chronological age alone.[43] However, statin therapy is associated with side effects including myalgias, myopathy, muscle weakness, injuries, and arthropathies.[44] Statins have also been associated with cognitive dysfunction, which may further contribute to reduced functional status, increased risk of falls, and further disability.[42]

MICROVASCULAR COMPLICATIONS

The risk of microvascular complications is generally proportional to the duration of diabetes.

Good control of diabetes is an effective means of reducing the progress of diabetic microvascular complications.[45,46]

- *Diabetic nephropathy*: It is characterized by increased quantities of albumin, diabetic glomerular lesions, and a decrease of GFR, which ultimately may lead to renal failure. T2DM is the leading cause of end-stage renal disease.
- *Microalbuminuria*: It is defined as albumin excretion rate of 30–300 mg/24 h and is an early manifestation of diabetic nephropathy. The presence or absence of albuminuria should therefore be routinely tested. If present, the use of angiotensin-converting enzyme (ACE) inhibitors and angiotensin receptor blocking agents have been found to slow down the rate of progression of renal dysfunction.[47-49] Early referral to a nephrologist is suggested for patients who have an established kidney disease due to diabetes.
- *Diabetic retinopathy*: An annual fundus examination by an eye disease specialist is recommended for all patients with T2DM after 5 years of diabetes and the elderly are no exception to this rule. Needless to add that the diagnostic and therapeutic recommendations of the specialist should be followed.
- *Diabetic neuropathy*: It is the most common complication of diabetes affecting as many as 50% of patients with T1DM and T2DM.[50] It is a potentially serious complication of diabetes, which can lead to foot ulceration, infections, and amputations. Elderly are at increased risk for lower extremity amputations. The patients should be educated about the care of their feet and a detailed foot examination including the neurological examination should be conducted at least once a year.

The most common type of neuropathy in diabetes is the "peripheral neuropathy". Patients frequently complain of numbness and tingling in their hands, more often in their feet. This may ultimately result in loss of sensation, leading to foot injury of which the patients may not be aware of. A combination of loss of sensation and decreased vascular supply may ultimately lead to partial amputations of the lower extremities.

Autonomic neuropathy may result in organ dysfunction, manifesting as gastroparesis, anhidrosis, diarrhea, bladder dysfunction, and erectile dysfunction in men.

Cardiovascular manifestations of autonomic neuropathy may result in resting tachycardia, decrease exercise tolerance, silent ischemia, and even sudden death. Cardiovascular autonomic dysfunction is associated with increased risk of silent myocardial ischemia and increased mortality.

There is no specific treatment for diabetic neuropathy. Several drugs have been used for pain control including gabapentin, pregabalin, amitriptyline, and duloxetine with varying degree of success.[51]

CONCLUSION

Diabetes and prediabetes are both very common in the elderly population. Since prediabetes and diabetes are both associated with increased risk for CVD and the rate of progression of prediabetes to diabetes can be potentially slowed down, it is recommended that elderly population undergo routine screening for diabetes. Lifestyle modification, namely exercise for 150 minutes a week, has been shown to significantly slow down the rate of progression of prediabetes to diabetes and is more effective in the elderly as compared to younger age groups.

Cardiovascular complications (both micro- and macrovascular) are a major cause of morbidity and mortality in diabetes and the elderly seems to be more susceptible to these complications. Besides diabetes, hypertension, and hyperlipidemia are major risk factors for these complications. Therefore, every effort should be made to control hyperglycemia, hypertension, and reduce the level of lipids, particularly LDL-C. However, there are many complicating factors in the elderly that may affect the overall management. An overall health assessment therefore, must be performed and individualized targets for the control of hyperglycemia, blood pressure, and lipids must be arrived at by shared decision-making. The ultimate goal of the management plan should be to improve the functional status of the patient and minimizing the complications.

REFERENCES

1. Saeedi P, Petersohn I, Salpea P, Malanda B, Karuranga S, Unwin N, et al. Global and regional diabetes prevalence estimates for 2019 and projections for 2030 and 2045: Results from the International Diabetes Federation Diabetes Atlas, 9th edition. Diabetes Res Clin Pract. 2019;157:107843.
2. International Diabetes Federation (IDF). (2019). Diabetes prevalence (% of population ages 20 to 79). [online] Available from data.worldbank.org/indicator/sh.sta.diab.zs. [Last accessed April, 2020].
3. Centers for Disease Control and Prevention (CDC). (2020). National Diabetes Statistics Report 2020: Estimates of Diabetes and its Burden in the United

States. [online] Available from cdc.gov/diabetes/pdfs/data/statistics/national-diabetes-statistics-report.pdf. [Last accessed April, 2020].
4. Statista. (2019). Share of old age population (65 years and older) in the total U.S. population from 1950 to 2050. [online] Available from statista.com/statistics/457822/share-of-old-age-population-in-the-total-us-population/. [Last accessed April, 2020].
5. Centers for Disease Control and Prevention (CDC). (2011). National Diabetes Fact Sheet, 2011: Data Sources, Methods, and References for Estimates of Diabetes and Prediabetes. [online] Available from https://www.cdc.gov/diabetes/pubs/pdf/methods11.pdf. [Last accessed April, 2020].
6. Rizvi AA. Management of Diabetes in Older Adults. Am J Med Sci. 2007;333:35-47.
7. LeRoith D, Biessels GJ, Braithwaite SS, Casanueva FF, Draznin B, Halter JB, et al. Treatment of Diabetes in Older Adults: An Endocrine Society* Clinical Practice Guideline. J Clin Endocrinol Metab. 2019;104:1520-74.
8. Halter JB, Musi N, McFarland Horne F, Crandall JP, Goldberg A, Harkless L, et al. Diabetes and cardiovascular disease in older adults: current status and future directions. Diabetes. 2014;63:2578-89.
9. Diabetes Prevention Program Research Group. Changes in albumin excretion in the diabetes prevention program. Diabetes Care. 2009;32:720-5.
10. DECODE Study Group, the European Diabetes Epidemiology Group. Glucose tolerance and cardiovascular mortality: comparison of fasting and 2-hour diagnostic criteria. Arch Intern Med. 2001;161:397-405.
11. Gossain VV, Aldasouqi S. The challenge of undiagnosed prediabetes, diabetes and associated cardiovascular disease. Int J Diabetes Mellitus. 2010;2:43-6.
12. Unwin N, Shaw J, Zimmet P, Alberti KG. Impaired glucose tolerance and impaired fasting glycaemia: the current status on definition and intervention. Diabet Med. 2002;19:708-23.
13. Alberti KG, Zimmet P, Shaw J. International Diabetes Federation: a consensus on Type 2 diabetes prevention. Diabet Med. 2007;24:451-63.
14. Knowler WC, Barrett-Connor E, Fowler SE, Hamman RF, Lachin JM, Walker EA, et al. Reduction in the incidence of type 2 diabetes with lifestyle intervention or metformin. N Engl J Med. 2002;346:393-403.
15. Apolzan JW, Venditti EM, Edelstein SL, Knowler WC, Dabelea D, Boyko EJ, et al. Long-Term Weight Loss With Metformin or Lifestyle Intervention in the Diabetes Prevention Program Outcomes Study. Ann Intern Med. 2019;170:682-90.
16. Haw JS, Galaviz KI, Straus AN, Kowalski AJ, Magee MJ, Weber MB, et al. Long-term Sustainability of Diabetes Prevention Approaches: A Systematic Review and Meta-analysis of Randomized Clinical Trials. JAMA Intern Med. 2017;177:1808-17.
17. Huang ES, Gorawara-Bhat R, Chin MH. Self-reported goals of older patients with type 2 diabetes mellitus. J Am Geriatr Soc. 2005;53:306-11.
18. Kimbro LB, Mangione CM, Steers WN, Duru OK, McEwen L, Karter A, et al. Depression and all-cause mortality in persons with diabetes mellitus: are older adults at higher risk? Results from the Translating Research Into Action for Diabetes Study. J Am Geriatr Soc. 2014;62:1017-22.
19. American Diabetes Association. Introduction: Standards of Medical Care in Diabetes—2020. Diabetes Care. 2020;43:S152-16.
20. Owens DK, Davidson KW, Krist AH, Barry MJ, Cabana M, Caughey AB, et al. Screening for Abdominal Aortic Aneurysm: US Preventive Services Task Force Recommendation Statement. JAMA. 2019;322: 2211-8.
21. American Diabetes Association. 8. Obesity Management for the Treatment of Type 2 Diabetes: Standards of Medical Care in Diabetes—2020. Diabetes Care. 2020;43:S89-97.
22. Park SW, Goodpaster BH, Strotmeyer ES, de Rekeneire N, Harris TB, Schwartz AV, et al. Decreased muscle strength and quality in older adults with type 2 diabetes: the health, aging, and body composition study. Diabetes. 2006;55:1813-8.

23. Park SW, Goodpaster BH, Strotmeyer ES, Kuller LH, Broudeau R, Kammerer C, et al. Accelerated loss of skeletal muscle strength in older adults with type 2 diabetes: the health, aging, and body composition study. Diabetes Care. 2007;30:1507-12.
24. Villareal DT, Chode S, Parimi N, Sinacore DR, Hilton T, Armamento-Villareal R, et al. Weight loss, exercise, or both and physical function in obese older adults. N Engl J Med. 2011;364:1218-29.
25. Evert AB, Dennison M, Gardner CD, Garvey WT, Lau KHK, MacLeod J, et al. Nutrition Therapy for Adults With Diabetes or Prediabetes: A Consensus Report. Diabetes Care. 2019;42:731-54.
26. Wylie C, Copeman J, Kirk SFL. Health and social factors affecting the food choice and nutritional intake of elderly people with restricted mobility. J Hum Nutr Dietet. 1999;12:375-80.
27. Trichopoulou A, Orfanos P, Norat T, Bueno-de-Mesquita B, Ocké MC, Peeters PH, et al. Modified Mediterranean diet and survival: EPIC-elderly prospective cohort study. BMJ. 2005;330:991.
28. Garber AJ, Handelsman Y, Grunberger G, Einhorn D, Abrahamson MJ, Barzilay JI, et al. Consensus Statement by the American Association of Clinical Endocrinologists and American College of Endocrinology on the comprehensive type 2 diabetes management algorithm—2020 Executive Summary. Endocr Pract. 2020;26:107-39.
29. Lee PG, Jackson EA, Richardson CR. Exercise Prescriptions in Older Adults. Am Fam Physician. 2017;95:425-32.
30. Feinkohl I, Aung PP, Keller M, Robertson CM, Morling JR, McLachlan S, et al. Severe hypoglycemia and cognitive decline in older people with type 2 diabetes: the Edinburgh type 2 diabetes study. Diabetes Care. 2014;37:507-15.
31. Lee AK, Rawlings AM, Lee CJ, Gross AL, Huang ES, Sharrett AR, et al. Severe hypoglycaemia, mild cognitive impairment, dementia and brain volumes in older adults with type 2 diabetes: the Atherosclerosis Risk in Communities (ARIC) cohort study. Diabetologia. 2018;61:1956-65.
32. Goto A, Arah OA, Goto M, Terauchi Y, Noda M. Severe hypoglycaemia and cardiovascular disease: systemic review and meta-analysis with bias analysis. BMJ. 2013;347:f4533.
33. Hanefeld M, Frier BM, Pistrosch F. Hypoglycemia and Cardiovascular Risk: Is There a Major Link? Diabetes Care. 2016;39:S205-9.
34. Bell KJ, Barclay AW, Petocz P, Colagiuri S, Brand-Miller JC. Efficacy of carbohydrate counting in type 1 diabetes: a systemic review and meta-analysis. Lancet Diabetes Endocrinol. 2014;2:133-40.
35. American Diabetes Association. 9. Pharmacologic Approaches to Glycemic Treatment: Standards of Medical Care in Diabetes-2020. Diabetes Care. 2020;43:S98-110.
36. American Diabetes Association. 10. Cardiovascular Disease and Risk Management: Standards of Medical Care in Diabetes—2020. Diabetes Care. 2020;43:S111-34.
37. de Boer IH, Bangalore S, Benetos A, Davis AM, Michos ED, Muntner P, et al. Diabetes and Hypertension: A Position Statement by the American Diabetes Association. Diabetes Care. 2017;40:1273-84.
38. Ettehad D, Emdin CA, Kiran A, Anderson SG, Callender T, Emberson J, et al. Blood pressure lowering for prevention of cardiovascular disease and death: a systematic review and meta-analysis. Lancet. 2016;387:957-67.
39. Grundy SM, Stone NJ, Bailey AL, Beam C, Birtcher KK, Blumenthal RS, et al. 2018 AHA/ACC/AACVPR/AAPA/ABC/ACPM/ADA/AGS/APhA/ASPC/NLA/PCNA Guideline on the Management of Blood Cholesterol: A Report of the American College of Cardiology/American Heart Association Task Force on Clinical Practice Guidelines. J Am Coll Cardiol. 2019;139:e1046-81.
40. Lloyd SM, Stott DJ, de Craen AJ, Kearney PM, Sattar N, Perry I, et al. Long-term effects of statin treatment in elderly people: extended follow-up of the PROspective Study of Pravastatin in the Elderly at Risk (PROSPER). PLoS One. 2013;8:e72642.

41. Han BH, Sutin D, Williamson JD, Davis BR, Piller LB, Pervin H, et al. Effect of Statin Treatment vs Usual Care on Primary Cardiovascular Prevention Among Older Adults: The ALLHAT-LLT Randomized Clinical Trial. JAMA Intern Med. 2017;177:955-65.
42. Curfman G. Risk of statin therapy in older adults. JAMA Intern Med. 2017;177:966.
43. Strandberg TE. Role of Stain Therapy in Primary Prevention of Cardiovascular Disease in Elderly Patients. Curr Atheroscler Rep. 2019;21:28.
44. Mansi I, Frei CR, Pugh MJ, Makris U, Mortensen EM. Statins and musculoskeletal conditions, arthropathies, and injuries. JAMA Intern Med. 2013;173:1-10.
45. Brown JS, Wing R, Barrett-Connor E, Nyberg LM, Kusek JW, Orchard TJ, et al. Lifestyle intervention is associated with lower prevalence of urinary incontinence: the Diabetes Prevention Program. Diabetes Care. 2006;29:385-90.
46. Intensive blood-glucose control with sulphonylureas or insulin compared with conventional treatment and risk of complication in patients with type 2 diabetes (UKPDS 33). UK Prospective Diabetes Study (UKPDS) Group. Lancet. 1998;352:837-53.
47. Lewis EJ, Hunsicker LG, Bain RP, Rohde RD. The effect of angiotensin-converting-enzyme inhibition on diabetic nephropathy. The Collaborative Study Group. N Engl J Med. 1993;329:1456-62.
48. Lewis EJ, Hunsicker LG, Clarke WR, Berl T, Pohl MA, Lewis BJ, et al. Renoprotective effect of the angiotensin-receptor antagonist irbesartan in patients with nephropathy due to type 2 diabetes. N Engl J Med. 2001;345:851-60.
49. Barnett AH, Bain SC, Bouter P, Karlberg B, Madsbad S, Jervell J, et al. Angiotensin-receptor blockade versus converting-enzyme inhibition in type 2 diabetes and nephropathy. N Engl J Med. 2004;351:1952-61.
50. Quan D, Khardori R. (2020). Diabetic Neuropathy. [online] Available from https://emedicine.medscape.com/article/1170337-overview. [Last accessed April, 2020].
51. American Diabetes Association. 11. Microvascular Complications and Foot Care: Standards of Medical Care in Diabetes-2020. Diabetes Care. 2020;43:S135-51.

Index

Page numbers followed by *f* refer to figure, *fc* refer to flowchart, and *t* refer to table.